VIVA VOCE *for* BDS Ist Year Students

Anatomy, Physiology, Biochemistry & Dental Anatomy and Histology

More than 1500 Questions & Answers Covered

Editors

Mahindra Kumar Anand
MBBS MS DO PhD
Professor and Head
Department of Anatomy
Sudha Rustagi College of Dental Sciences and Research
Kheri More, Faridabad, Haryana, India
Visting Professor
University of West Indies, Cave Hill Campus, Barbados, West Indies

Uma Gaur
MBBS MS
Professor, Department of Anatomy
Lady Hardinge Medical College, New Delhi, India

JAYPEE BROTHERS MEDICAL PUBLISHERS (P) LTD

New Delhi • Panama City • London

Published by
Jaypee Brothers Medical Publishers (P) Ltd

Corporate Office
4838/24, Ansari Road, Daryaganj, **New Delhi** 110 002, India
Phone: +91-11-43574357, Fax: +91-11-43574314
Website: www.jaypeebrothers.com

Offices in India

- **Ahmedabad**, e-mail: ahmedabad@jaypeebrothers.com
- **Bengaluru**, e-mail: bangalore@jaypeebrothers.com
- **Chennai**, e-mail: chennai@jaypeebrothers.com
- **Delhi**, e-mail: jaypee@jaypeebrothers.com
- **Hyderabad**, e-mail: hyderabad@jaypeebrothers.com
- **Kochi**, e-mail: kochi@jaypeebrothers.com
- **Kolkata**, e-mail: kolkata@jaypeebrothers.com
- **Lucknow**, e-mail: lucknow@jaypeebrothers.com
- **Mumbai**, e-mail: mumbai@jaypeebrothers.com
- **Nagpur**, e-mail: nagpur@jaypeebrothers.com

Overseas Offices

- **Central America Office, Panama City, Panama**, Ph: 001-507-317-0160
  e-mail: cservice@jphmedical.com, Website: www.jphmedical.com
- **Europe Office, UK**, Ph: +44 (0) 2031708910
  e-mail: info@jpmedpub.com

VIVA VOCE for BDS Ist Year Students

Fist Edition: 2011

ISBN 978-93-5025-425-7

Typeset at JPBMP typesetting unit

Printed in India

List of Contributors

Geetika Juneja BDS
Faridabad, Haryana, India

Manisha Arora MSC, D Phil (Biochemistry)
Professor
Department of Biochemistry
Muzaffarnagar Medical College and Hospital
Muzaffarnagar, UP, India

Mital Patel MBBS, MS (Anatomy)
Associate Professor
Department of Anatomy
MP Shah Medical College
Jam Nagar, Gujarat, India

Prasoon Shukla BDS, MDS (Prosthodontics)
Sr. Lecturer
Department of Prosthodontics
Sudha Rustagi College of Dental
Sciences and Research
Faridabad, Haryana, India

Shivani Sharma MBBS, MD (Physiology)
Assistant Professor
Department of Physiology
Muzaffarnagar Medical College and Hospital
Muzaffarnagar, UP, India

TC Singel MBBS, MS (Anatomy)
Professor and Head
Department of Anatomy
MP Shah Medical College
Jam Nagar, Gujarat, India

Uma Gaur MBBS, MS
Professor, Department of Anatomy
Lady Hardinge Medical College
New Delhi, India

Vishal Juneja BDS
Reader
Department of Dental Anatomy and Histology
Sudha Rustagi College of Dental
Sciences and Research
Faridabad, Haryana, India

Preface

Viva Voce forms an important part of the examination system all over the globe. Textbooks provide the basic knowledge and in-depth understanding of the subjects but it is often difficult for the students to translate the knowledge into answers in viva examinations in a short span of fifteen to twenty minutes. Hence, we have developed a consise and comprehensive viva voce book with important viva questions and their relevant answers to provide an overall review and quick revision before examinations.

The book has been designed primarily for dental students of first year and consists of important question from all subjects of the first year.

The questions are arrange section-wise and chapter-wise to provide better orientation of the subject and it would also enable the student to refer to the corresponding topic in their textbooks if required for further details.

I hope the students will find the contents useful for their examinations and enjoy reading this book.

Mahindra Kumar Anand
MBBS MS DO PhD

Uma Gaur
MBBS MS

From the Publisher's Desk

We request all the readers to provide us their valuable suggestions / errors (if any) at:
jaypeemcqproduction@gmail.com
so as to help us in further improvement of this book in the subsequent edition.

ACKNOWLEDGMENTS

We would like to acknowledge Mr Dharma Vir Gupta, Chairman, Lala Bhagwan Das Education Trust and Sudha Rustagi College of Dental Sciences and Research, for providing a conducive environment for my work. I also thank Prof. Neeraj Rampal, Principal, Sudha Rustagi College of Dental Sciences and Research, who provided consistent cooperation in the successful completion of this book. My sincere thanks to Mr. Deepak Gupta, Secretary, Lala Bhagwan Das Educational Trust and Sudha Rustagi College of Dental Sciences and Research for ensuring continuous support and encouragement.

We are grateful to the valuable contribution to the text of the book by Dr TC Singel, Dr Mital Patel, Dr Shivani Sharma, Dr Manisha Arora, Dr Vishal Juneja, Dr Prasoon Shukla, Dr Geetika Juneja.

Our sincere thanks to Shri Jitendar P Vij (Chairman and Managing Director) of M/s Jaypee Brothers Medical Publishers (P) Ltd., Mr Tarun Duneja, Director of Publishing and Mr Bupesh Arora (General Manager, Publishing) Jaypee Brothers Medical Publishers (P) Ltd., for their dedicated enthusiasm and help throughout writing of the book.

Mr Sudhir Sharma deserves special thanks for his excellent formatting in the making of manuscript of the book.

Mahindra Kumar Anand
MBBS MS DO PhD

Uma Gaur
MBBS MS

CONTENTS

SECTION 1—HUMAN ANATOMY 1-48

- General Anatomy 1
- Systemic Anatomy 6
- Head and Neck 11
- Neuroanatomy 34
- Genetics 37
- Histology 39
- Embryology 43

SECTION 2—PHYSIOLOGY 49-82

- General Physiology 49
- Nerve Muscle Physiology 51
- Blood 53
- Digestive System 57
- Cardiovascular System 60
- Respiratory System 63
- Excretory System 66
- Metabolism and Nutrition 68
- Nervous System 69
- Special Senses 72
- Endocrine System 76
- Reproductive System 80
- Skin and its Appendages 81

SECTION 3—BIOCHEMISTRY 83-97

- Carbohydrate Chemistry and Metabolism 83
- Amino Acid, Protein Chemistry and Metabolism 85
- Nucleic Acid Chemistry and Metabolism 87
- Lipid Chemistry and Metabolism 88
- Enzymes and Isoenzymes 90
- Biological Oxidation 91
- Acid-Base Balance 92
- Water and Electrolyte Balance 92
- Mineral Metabolism 93
- Detoxification 93
- Vitamins 94
- Chemical Composition of Teeth 96
- Biochemistry of Saliva 96
- Molecular Biochemistry 97

SECTION 4—DENTAL ANATOMY AND HISTOLOGY 98-108

- Dental Anatomy 98
- Dental Histology and Development 105

SECTION – 1

Human Anatomy

General Anatomy

Q.1. What is anatomical position and its importance?

Ans. Anatomical position: Body is erect, the eyes face forward, and arms are kept by the side with palms facing forward. The legs are kept together with feet directed forwards.

Importance of anatomical position: All structures of our body are described in relation to this position, irrespective to any body posture in space.

Q.2. Define lithotomy position?

Ans. Person lies supine with hips and knees semiflexed, thighs abducted and feet strapped.

Q.3. What are functions of cell membrane or plasma membrane?

Ans. Functions of plasma membrane

1. Maintains the shape of a cell.
2. It is selectively permeable to Na^+, K^+, Ca^{++}, Cl^- and HCO_3^- through special channels.
3. Amino acids, proteins, nucleic precursors pass through channels in the membrane, either actively or passively.
4. Lipid soluble substances pass through cell membrane.
5. Various receptors are present on the cell membrane.
6. It aids in recognition of identical cells with the help of cell coat which is specific to those cells.
7. It helps in endocytosis and exocytosis.

Q.4. What are the types of intercellular junctions?

Ans. Intercellular and extracellular matrix junctions are (Fig. 1.1):

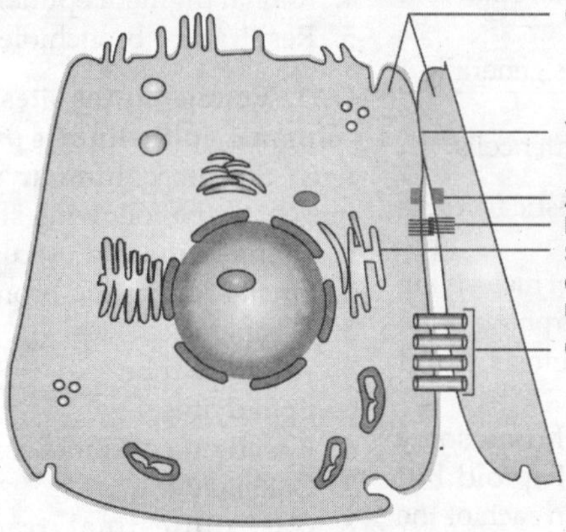

Fig. 1.1: Intercellular junctions

1. **Macula adherens (desmosome):** Intercellular gap of 25 nm bridged by filaments
2. **Zonula adherens:** Intercellular gap of 20 nm filled by adhesive non-stainable material, there are no filaments. These junctions are found in the apical region of epithelial, endothelial and mesothelial cells.
3. **Zonula occludens (tight junctions):** There is no intercellular gap and the membranes of adjacent cells come in close contact.
4. **Gap junction:** Intercellular gap of 3 nm traversed by numerous dense beats arranged in a hexagonal array.
5. **Fascia adherens:** It is similar to zonula adherens. It is present between smooth muscle cells and intercalated disks of cardiac muscle cells.
6. **Hemidesmosomes:** They are known as anchoring junctions between bases of epithelial cells and basal lamina.

Q.5. What are the different phases of cell cycle?

Ans. Cell cycle is the period extending from the formation of a cell from its parent cell to its own division that further gives rise to daughter cells. The cell cycle is divided into four phases. These phases are as follows (Fig. 1.2):

1. G_1–phase
2. S–phase
3. G_2–phase
4. M–phase

Q.6. What are the characteristic features of mitosis?

Ans. Characteristic features of mitosis are

1. Chromosome number remains same in daughter cells as in the parent cell.
2. Mitosis is preceded by DNA synthesis in S-phase and the dividing cell becomes tetraploid with each chromosome consisting of two identical strands known as chromatids.

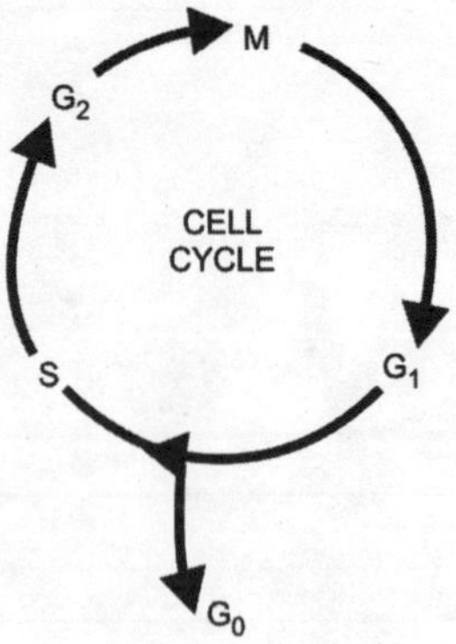

Fig. 1.2: Cell cycle

3. It is responsible for the growth of an individual and helps in the repair and replacement of old cells.
4. The duration of mitosis is generally 1 to 2 hours.
5. Mitosis results in 2 daughter cells.

Q.7. What are the characteristic features of meiosis?

Ans. Characteristic features of meiosis are

1. There is a very short interphase or no interphase between meiosis I and meiosis II.
2. During meiosis I the chromosome number is reduced to haploid but DNA content is diploid in each of the two resultant cells.
3. After meiosis II, the daughter cells have haploid (n) number of chromosomes and haploid DNA. This ultimately helps to restore diploid (2n) number of chromosomes after fertilization.
4. There is exchange of genetic material between the homologous chromosomes in meiosis I
5. The duration of meiosis is 24 days in males and it lasts for many years in females.
6. Meiosis results in 4 daughter cells.

Q.8. Enumerate different types of epithelium.

Ans. Various types of epithelium are:

1. Simple squamous epithelium
2. Simple columnar epithelium
3. Simple cuboidal epithelium
4. Stratified squamous epithelium
5. Stratified columnar epithelium
6. Stratified cuboidal epithelium
7. Pseudostratified columnar epithelium
8. Transitional epithelium.

Q.9. Where do you find simple squamous epithelium?

Ans. Simple squamous epithelium is present at the following sites:

1. Blood vessels
2. Alveoli
3. Bowman's capsule
4. Peritoneum
5. Pleura.

Q.10. Enumerate the sites where simple cuboidal epithelium is present?

Ans. Simple cuboidal epithelium is found at the following sites:

1. Thyroid follicles
2. Small ducts of digestive glands
3. Germinal epithelium of ovary
4. Retinal pigment epithelium
5. Respiratory bronchiole.

Q.11. Enumerate the sites where simple columnar epithelium is present?

Ans. Simple columnar epithelium is present at the following sites:

1. Uterine tube and uterus
2. Small bronchi and bronchioles
3. Tympanic cavities
4. Auditory tube
5. Epididymis
6. Ependyma of spinal cord
7. Gallbladder
8. Gastrointestinal tract (Stomach, duodenum, jejunum, ileum, colon, rectum).

Q.12. Where do you find pseudostratified ciliated columnar epithelium

Ans. Pseudostratified ciliated columnar epithelium is present in

1. Trachea
2. Bronchi
3. Ductus deferens
4. Male urethra.

Q.13. Where do you find nonkeratinized stratified squamous epithelium?

Ans. Nonkeratinized stratified squamous epithelium is present at the following sites:

1. Oral cavity
2. Tongue
3. Tonsils
4. Pharynx
5. Esophagus
6. Vagina
7. External urethral orifice
8. Cornea
9. Conjunctiva.

Q.14. Enumerate the sites where stratified cuboidal epithelium is present?

Ans. Stratified cuboidal epithelium is present at:

1. Ducts of sweat glands and mammary gland
2. Seminiferous tubules
3. Ovarian follicles.

Q.15. Where do you find stratified columnar epithelium?

Ans. Stratified columnar epithelium is found at the following sites:

1. Fornix of conjunctiva
2. Anal mucous membrane
3. Urethra.

Q.16. Where do you find transitional epithelium?

Ans. Transitional epithelium is present at the following sites:

1. Pelvis of kidney
2. Ureter
3. Urinary bladder
4. Urethra.

Q.17. Enumerate cells present in connective tissue.

Ans. Two types of cells are present in connective tissues

1. Resident cells namely, fibroblasts, adipocytes and mesenchymal stem cells
2. Migrant cells: These are derived from blood circulation and consist of macrophages or histocytes, plasma cells, mast cells, pigment cells , lymphocytes and monocytes.

Q.18. What are the functions of connective tissue?

Ans. Functions of connective tissue are:

1. Binds together various structures.
2. Facilitates passage of neurovascular bundle.
3. In the form of deep fascia, connective tissue keeps the muscles and tendons in position, gives origin to muscles and forms different functional compartment of muscles.
4. In the form of ligaments, bind the bones.
5. Attaches muscle to the bone with the help of tendons and facilitates a concentrated pull.
6. Facilitates venous return in lower limb with the help of deep fascia.
7. Helps in wound repair due to the presence of fibroblasts.

Q.19. Define bursa.

Ans. It is a sac of synovial membrane supported by dense irregular connective tissue. It helps to reduce friction. Hence, it is found at those places where two structures which move relative to each other in tight apposition. Bursae present at different places are:

1. Subcutaneous bursa—Between skin and bone.
2. Submuscular bursa—Between muscle and bone.
3. Subfascial bursa—Between fascia and bone.
4. Interligamentous bursa—The bursa between two ligaments.

Q.20. What is adventitious bursa?

Ans. Adventitious bursa develops over bony parts which are subjected to much friction or pressure. It develops due to physiological reasons and is not present normally, e.g., Tailor's ankle, Porter's shoulder, Weaver's bottom.

Q.21. Name the types of bones in the body?

Ans. According to shape, ossification and presence of cavity, bones are classified as follows:

1. Long bone
2. Short bone
3. Flat bone
4. Irregular bone
5. Pneumatic bone
6. Sesamoid bone
7. Accessory bone

Q.22. Give examples of pneumatic bones.

Ans. Maxilla, sphenoid, ethmoid and squamous part of frontal bone.

Q.23. What is a sesamoid bone?

Ans. These bones develop in the tendon of a muscle. They share the load of the tendon and change the direction of pull of the tendon. Periosteum is absent in these bones. Examples, patella, pisiform, fabella.

Q.24. What is arterial supply of a long bone?

Ans. A long bone is supplied by 4 sets of arteries namely (Fig. 1.3).

1. Nutrient artery
2. Metaphyseal arteries
3. Epiphyseal arteries
4. Periosteal arteries

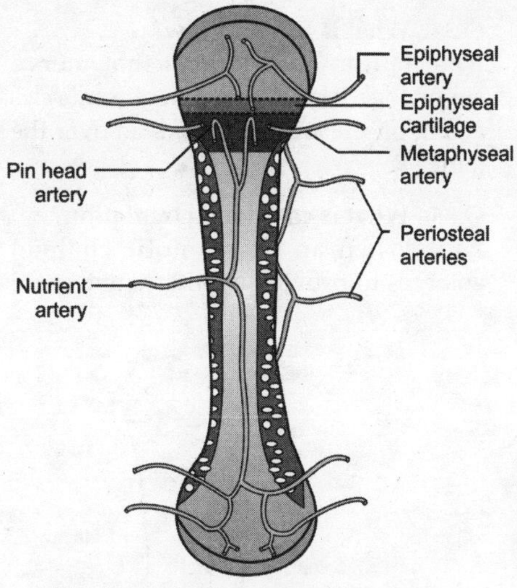

Fig. 1.3: Arterial supply of long bone

Q.25. What is the composition of a bone?

Ans. Bone is made up of 40% organic component and 60% inorganic component.

Organic component consists of type I collagen fibers with osteoblasts, osteoclasts and osteocytes.

Inorganic component contains calcium hydroxyapatite crystals Ca^{++} $(H_3O)_2 (PO_4)_6 (OH)_2$ with small amounts of magnesium, sodium and carbonate.

Q.26. What are characteristic features of cartilage?

Ans. Characteristic features of cartilage are:

1. Cartilage is avascular. It receives its nutrition through diffusion from the nearest capillaries.
2. Cartilage has no nerves. Hence it is insensitive to pain.
3. Cartilage is surrounded by perichondrium.
4. Cartilage grows by appositional as well as interstitial method of growth.
5. Cartilage has low antigenicity due to lack of lymphatics, homogeneous transplantation of cartilage is possible without much risk of rejection.

Q.27. What are different types of cartilages and their distribution?

Ans. Different types of cartilages:

1. **Hyaline cartilage**
   Distribution: Articular cartilage, thyroid cartilage, cricoid cartilage, lower part of arytenoid cartilage, tracheal rings, costal cartilages, bronchial cartilages, nasal cartilage.
2. **Elastic cartilage**
   Distribution: Pinna of external ear, epiglottis, corniculate and cuneiform cartilages, apex of arytenoid cartilage, auditory tube, external auditory meatus.
3. **White fibro-cartilage**
   Distribution: Intervertebral disk, interpubic disk, menisci of knee joint, articular disk of temporomandibular, sternoclavicular and inferior radio-ulnar joints, labra of glenoid and acetabulum.

Q.28. What are characteristics of skeletal muscle?

Ans. Characteristics of skeletal muscle are

1. It is the most abundant muscle in the body and is attached to the skeletal frame work.
2. It is supplied by spinal nerves. It is under voluntary control except muscles of pharynx and diaphragm.
3. Skeletal muscle fibers respond quickly to stimuli, undergo rapid contraction and get fatigued easily.
4. Skeletal musculature helps in adjusting the individual to his external environment.
5. Highest control of muscle activity is the cerebral cortex.
6. Histological sections of muscle fibers show cylindrical multi-nucleated fibers with cross striations seen under microscope.

Q.29. What are characteristics of smooth muscle?

Ans. Characteristics of smooth muscle are:

1. Smooth muscles surround the various viscera.
2. They are supplied by autonomic nervous system. They are less dependent on neuronal control.
3. They respond slowly to stimuli with a sustained contraction, do not fatigue easily.
4. They help in regulating internal environment.
5. Histological sections of muscle fibers show closely packed spindle shaped fibers with single central nucleus. Cross striations are not seen under microscope.

Q.30. What are characteristics of cardiac muscle?

ANATOMY

Ans. Characteristics of cardiac muscle are

1. Cardiac muscle forms the myocardium of heart.
2. Cardiac muscle is supplied by autonomic nervous system and has involuntary control.
3. Automatic and rhythmic contractions are seen in cardiac muscle. Nervous control is only to maintain the rhythm of cardiac muscle.
4. Histological sections show inter-connected cylindrical fibers joined by intercalated disks with fine striations.
5. The fibers of cardiac muscle function as a single mass, i.e. syncytium.

Q.31. What are different types of fibrous joint?

Ans. Types of fibrous joints:

1. Sutures (Fig. 1.4)
2. Syndesmosis (Fig. 1.5)
3. Gomphosis (Fig. 1.6)

Q.32. Give examples of secondary cartilaginous joints.

Ans. Manubriosternal joint, symphysis pubis, intervertebral disk.

Q.33. What are different types of synovial joint?

Ans. Different types of synovial joints are

1. **Plane joint,** e.g. Acromioclavicular joint.
2. **Uniaxial joint**
   - Hinge joint, e.g. Elbow joint.
   - Pivot joint, e.g. Superior radioulnar joint.
   - Condylar joint, e.g. Knee joint.
3. **Biaxial joint**
   - Ellipsoid joint, e.g. Wrist joint.
   - Saddle joint, e.g. Ist carpo-metacarpal joint.
4. **Polyaxial joint**
   - Ball and socket joint, e.g. shoulder joint.

Q.34. What is Hilton's law?

Ans. Hilton's law states that, nerve supplying a joint also supplies the muscles acting on the joint and the skin over the joint.

Q.35. What is collateral circulation?

Ans. When an anastomotic channel enlarges to provide an alternative route for circulation of blood following the interruption of flow in the primary artery it is known as collateral circulation. Collateral circulation develops rapidly in young people.

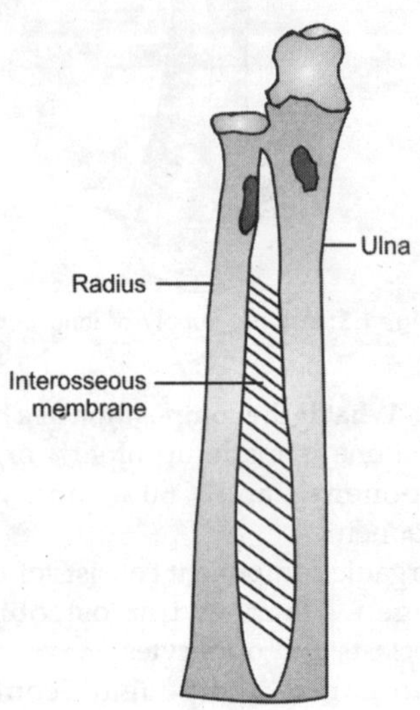

Fig. 1.5: Syndesmosis

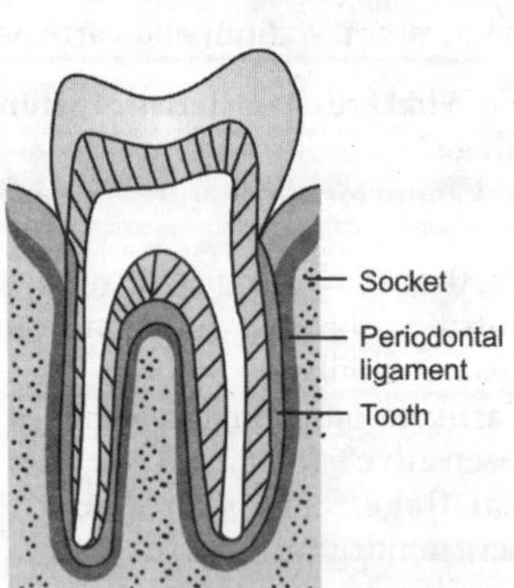

Fig. 1.6: Gomphosis

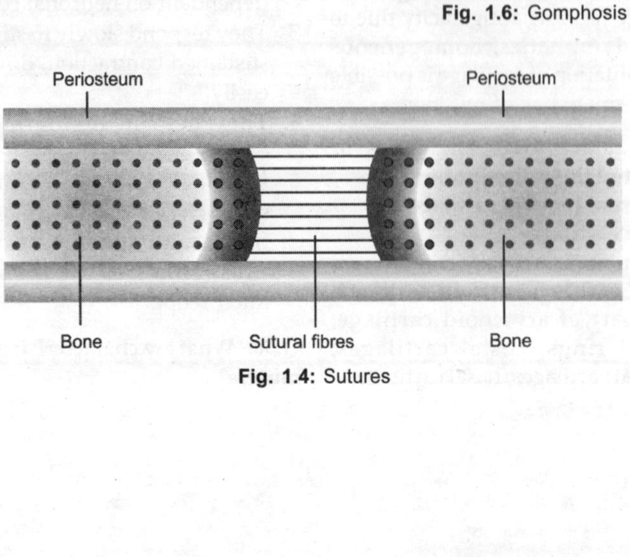

Fig. 1.4: Sutures

Q.36. How many spinal nerves are there in the body?

Ans. There are 31 pairs of spinal nerves. These are:

1. 8 Cervical spinal nerves
2. 12 Thoracic spinal nerves
3. 5 Lumbar spinal nerves
4. 5 Sacral spinal nerves
5. 1 Coccygeal spinal nerve.

Q.37. Enumerate the different layers of epidermis of skin?

Ans. Epidermis is divided into five layers. From deep to superficial, these are:

1. Stratum basale
2. Stratum spinosum
3. Stratum granulosum
4. Stratum lucidum
5. Stratum corneum.

Q.38. What is the largest round cell in the human body?

Ans. Ovum, its size is 120-140 μ.

Q.39. Enumerate the endocrine organs in the body?

Ans. Important endocrine glands in the body are (Fig. 1.7):

1. Pituitary gland (hypophysis-cerebri)
2. Pineal gland (epiphysis cerebri)
3. Thyroid glands
4. Parathyroid glands
5. Adrenals
6. Islets of Langerhans (pancreas)
7. Ovaries, in females
8. Testes, in males
9. Placenta, during pregnancy.

Q.40. What is anthropometry?

Ans. It is the study of variations in the dimensions and bodily proportions of various bones in different races and of variations with age and sex in a single race.

Q.41. Why is symphysis menti is not a true secondary cartilaginous joint?

Ans. The fusion of two halves of the mandible takes place at the age of 3 years. Therefore, it behaves like a primary cartilaginous joint.

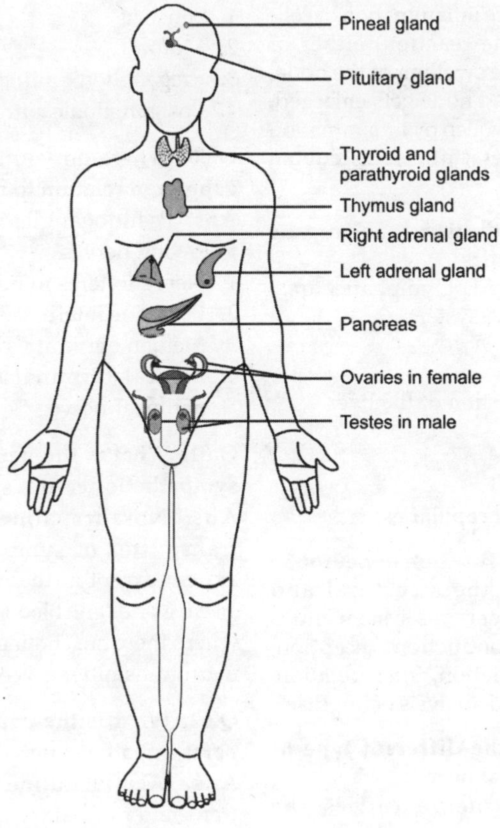

Fig. 1.7: Endocrine system

Q.42. What is the function of articular disk?

Ans. Articular disk performs the following functions:

1. It divides the joint cavity into two, this increases the range of movement.
2. It acts as shock absorber.
3. It deepens the joint cavity.

Q.43. Where does the nerve supply of a joint lie?

Ans. Nerve supply of a joint lies in the capsule of the joint and its ligaments. Articular cartilage is insensitive.

Q.44. What is Wolff's law?

Ans. Wolff's law states that osteogenesis is directly proportional to stress and strain.

Q.45. Enumerate the unpaired bones in the body?

Ans. Unpaired bones are:

1. Frontal
2. Occipital
3. Sphenoid
4. Ethmoid
5. Vomer
6. Mandible
7. Hyoid
8. Vertebrae
9. Sternum
10. Sacrum
11. Coccyx

Q.46. What is a dermatome?

Ans. It is the part of the skin supplied by a single spinal segment.

Q.47. What is law of union of epiphysis?

Ans. It states that the epiphyseal center which appears first, unites last and epiphyseal center which appears last unite first.

Q.48. Define aponeurosis?

Ans. It is a regular dense connective tissue associated with the attachment of muscles. It is made up of densely arranged collagen fibers.

Q.49. Name the areas of body which do not bear any hairs.

Ans. These are following:

1. Palms
2. Soles
3. Dorsal surfaces of distal phalanges
4. Umbilicus
5. Glans penis
6. Inner surface of the prepuce
7. Inner surfaces of the labia majora
8. Labia minora
9. Surfaces of the eyelids
10. Exposed margins of the lips.

Q.50. What are end arteries? Enumerate them?

Ans. End arteries are the arteries which do not have any anastomosis. Following are the end arteries:

1. Central artery of the retina. It is considered as an absolute end artery
2. Central branches of cerebral arteries
3. Splenic artery
4. Vasa-recta of the small gut
5. Coronary arteries (anatomically they are not end-arteries although functionally they behave like end-arteries)
6. Appendicular artery
7. Supraduodenal artery of Wilky
8. Metaphyseal arteries
9. Arcuate arteries of the kidney.

Q.51. What are the areas in the body devoid of capillaries?

Ans. Following are the areas devoid of capillaries:

1. Epidermis of the skin
2. Hair
3. Nails
4. Cornea of the eye
5. Lens
6. Articular hyaline cartilages.

Q.52. Where do you find arterio-venous anastomosis in the body?

Ans. Following are the sites of arterio-venous anastomosis:

1. Tip of nose
2. Lips
3. Eye-lids
4. Lobule of ear
5. Finger tips
6. Nail-beds.

Q.53. Which arteries are formed by union of other arteries?

Ans. Following arteries are formed by fusion of other two arteries:

1. Basilar artery, due to union of vertebral arteries
2. Anterior spinal artery, due to fusion of anterior spinal branches of vertebral arteries

3. Azygos arteries of the vagina due to anastomosis between the branches of uterine and vaginal arteries.

Q.54. Which large size artery is made up of only endothelium and where is it present?
Ans. Internal carotid artery in the cavernous sinus.

Q.55. Enumerate the valveless veins?
Ans. Following veins are valveless:
1. Superior vena cava and inferior vena cava
2. Pulmonary veins
3. Portal vein
4. Hepatic veins
5. Renal veins
6. Uterine veins
7. Ovarian veins
8. Cerebral veins
9. Spinal veins
10. Veins of spongy tissue of bone
11. Umbilical veins
12. Veins, less than 2 mm in diameter.

Q.56. How does the lymph node enlarge? What is the effect?
Ans. The cells of lymph node are responsible for filtering bacteria or antigens and induce inflammation or cell-mediated immune reaction, either of which can produce swelling of the node. Hence, the involved node gets enlarged. When nodes are swollen by inflammation or blocked by metastatic cells, edema occurs.

Q.57. Enumerate the tissues and organs devoid of lymphatics?
Ans. Organs devoid of lymphatics are:
1. Central nervous system
2. Bone marrow
3. Eye ball
4. Intralobular portion of the liver
5. Internal ear
6. Red pulp of spleen
7. Fetal-placenta
8. Areas devoid of capillaries.

Q.58. What is the function of neuron?
Ans. Neuron is the structural and functional unit of nervous system and is responsible for conduction, reception, integration, association, interpretation, transformation and analysis of impulses.

Q.59. What are the different type of fibers in peripheral nerve?
Ans. Peripheral nerve carries the following fibers
1. Sensory
2. Motor
3. Preganglionic autonomic
4. Postganglionic autonomic

Q.60. Where do you find the pseudoganglia in relation to nerves?
Ans. Pseudoganglia are present with following nerves.
1. Nerve to teres minor muscle
2. Posterior interosseous nerve
3. Median nerve at wrist
4. Lateral terminal branch of deep peroneal nerve.

Q.61. What is the neurotransmitter of sympathetic nervous system?
Ans. Noradrenaline is the neurotransmitter of sympathetic nervous system except at the nerve endings for sweat glands and blood vessels of muscles where there are cholinergic neurons and neurotransmitter is acetylcholine.

Q.62. What is the neurotransmitter of parasympathetic nervous system?
Ans. Acetylcholine is the neurotransmitter of parasympathetic nervous system.

Systemic Anatomy

Q.63. What is skeletal system?
Ans. Skeletal system is composed of skeleton made up of bones which provide the basic structure to the body.

Q.64. What is axial skeleton?
Ans. It consists of skull, vertebral column, thoracic cage and hyoid bone.

Q.65. What is appendicular skeleton?
Ans. It consists of bones of upper and lower limbs

Bones forming upper limb skeleton are clavicle, scapula, humerus, radius, ulna, 8 carpal bones: scaphoid, lunate, triquetral, pisiform, trapezium, trapezoid, capitate, hamate, 5 metacarpals and 14 phalanges.

Bones forming lower limb skeleton: ilium, ischium, pubis, femur, patella, tibia, fibula, 8 tarsal bones: talus, calcaneum, navicular, cuboid and three cuneiform bones 5 metatarsals, 14 phalanges.

Q.66. What are the functions of skeleton?
Ans. (Fig. 1.8)
1. Skeleton forms the structural framework of the body.
2. It supports the body.
3. It transmits the weight of the body.
4. Bones and joints act as a biochemical levers on which muscles act to produce motion.
5. Skeleton of head and vertebral column protect the vital organs namely brain and spinal cord.
6. Skeletal frame work of thoracic cage (ribs and sternum) provides for the respiratory movements and protects the heart and lungs.
7. Bones serve as a reservoir of ions (Ca^{++}, PO_4, CO_3^-) in the mineral homeostasis of the body.
8. Bone marrow in adults is the source of red blood cells, granular white blood cells and platelets.
9. Cartilage is a precursor for bone formation. Most of the bones are laid down on cartilage. It also provides structural support in areas like ear, larynx and trachea where rigidity is not require.

Q.67. What are the types of muscles present in human body?
Ans. Muscle are divided into three types based on their location in relation to various body parts and on the differences in microscopic structure.
1. Skeletal muscle
2. Smooth muscle
3. Cardiac muscle

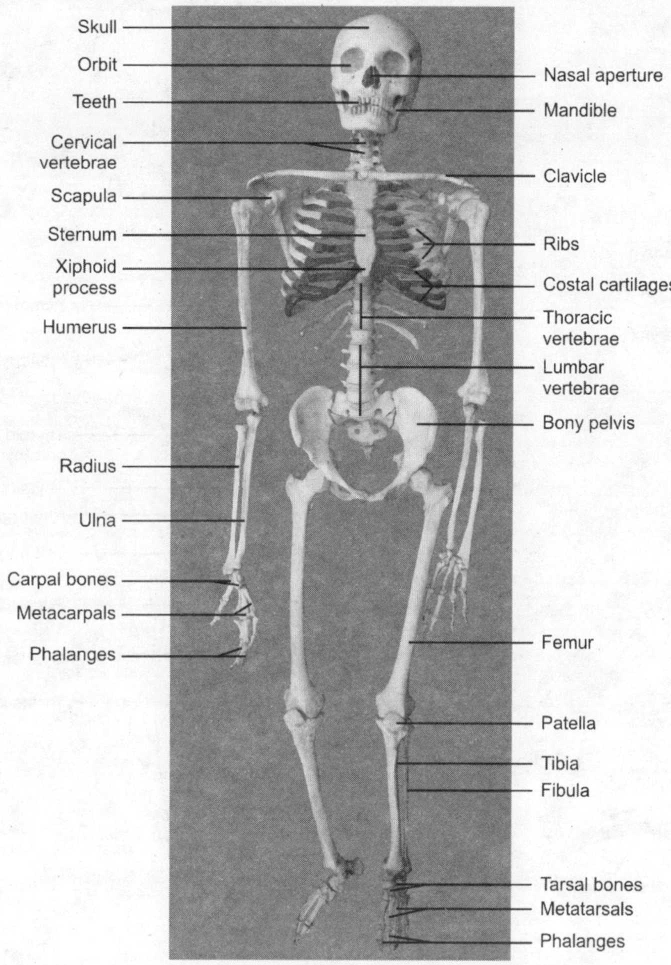

Fig. 1.8: Human skeleton (Skeleton system)

Q.68. What are the parts of respiratory system?

Ans. It consists of the following parts (Fig. 1.9):

1. **Upper respiratory tract**: Nose and paranasal sinuses, pharynx, larynx, trachea with two principal bronchi
2. **Lower respiratory tract** consisting of bronchopulmonary tree on each side with two lungs enclosed in pleura.

Musculo-skeletal framework of thorax enclosing the lungs and pleura is made up of thoracic cage, intercostal muscles and diaphragm.

Q.69. Name the muscles of inspiration?

Ans.

1. External intercostal muscles
2. Diaphragm
3. Accessory muscles: Erector spinae, scalene group of muscles, sternocleidomastoid, pectoralis major, serratus anterior, quadratus lumborum.

Q.70. Name the muscles of expiration?

Ans. Expiration is passive and occurs due to recoil of lungs. In forced expiration following muscles are involved:

1. Anterior abdominal wall muscles namely, rectus abdominis, internal oblique and transverse abdominis
2. Internal intercostal muscles

Q.71. What are the components of lymphatic system?

Ans. (Fig. 1.10)

1. Lymph and lymph vessels namely, lymph capillaries, lymph vessels proper and terminal lymph ducts (trunks)
2. Lymphoid tissue and lymphoid organs
   a. Primary lymphatic follicles
   b. Lymph nodes
   c. Spleen
   d. Thymus
   e. Bone marrow
   f. Mucosa associated lymphoid tissue

Q.72. What are the parts of excretory system?

Ans. The excretory function of the body is primarily carried out by a pair of kidneys. Kidneys are responsible for the filtration of blood and removal of waste substances like urea, creatinine, uric acid and others from the body. The filtrate undergoes a process of reabsorption and secretion which results in the formation of urine. The urine is carried from the kidneys to the **urinary bladder** by the **ureters** and is expelled to exterior during micturition through **urethra**. Kidneys, ureters, urinary bladder and urethra form the **urinary system**. This system helps in regulating the solute and water content of the body there by, regulating the composition and volume of extracellular fluid.

The other excretory organs of the body are skin (produces sweat), GIT (excretes faeces), respiratory tract (excretes CO_2) (Fig. 1.11).

Q.73. Name the parts of male reproductive system.

Ans. It consists of the following parts (Fig. 1.12):

1. Penis
2. Scrotum
3. Testes
4. Epididymis
5. Spermatic cord
6. Ductus deferens
7. Seminal vesicles
8. Ejaculatory duct
9. Prostate gland

First five form external genitalia of male.

Q.74. Name the parts of female reproductive system.

Ans. The female reproductive system consists of:

1. **External genitalia (Fig 1.14):** Female external genitalia is also known as vulva. It includes.
   a. Mons pubis
   b. Labia majora
   c. Labia minora
   d. Vestibule
   e. Hymen
   f. Clitoris

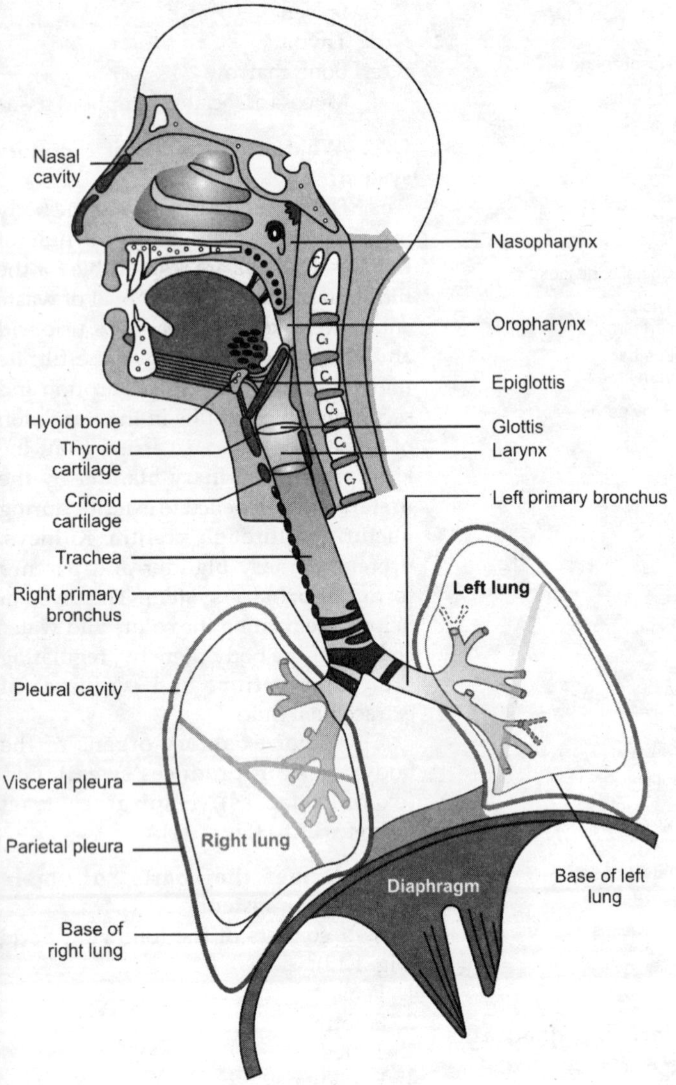

Fig. 1.9: Respiratory system

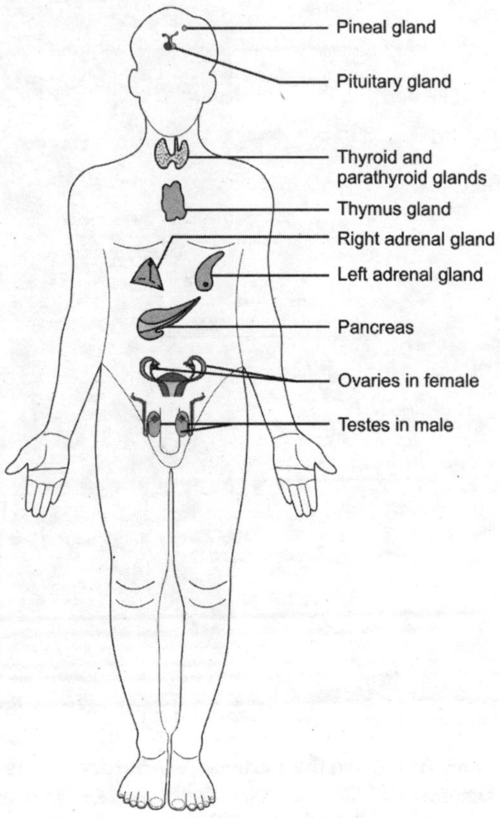

Fig. 1.10: Lymphatic system

   g. Bulb of the vestibule
   h. Greater vestibular glands (Bartholin's gland)
   i. Vaginal orifice
2. **Internal genitalia (Fig. 1.13)**
   a. Uterus and cervix
   b. A pair of fallopian tubes
   c. Vagina
   d. Two ovaries

Q.75. Name the parts of cardiovasulcar system?

Ans. (Fig. 1.15)

1. Heart
2. Large arteries: aorta, left common carotid artery, right common carotid artery, left external carotid artery, right external carotid artery, left internal carotid artery, right internal carotid artery, left and right subclavian arteries, left and right axillary arteries, left and right common iliac arteries, left and right internal iliac arteries, left and right external iliac arteries, left and right femoral arteries, left and right popliteal arteries.
3. *Medium and small arteries:* Right and left brachial arteries, Right and left radial arteries, Right and left ulnar arteries, Right and left posterior interosseous arteries, Right and left anterior interosseous arteries, left and right peroneal arteries, left and right anterior tibial arteries, left and right posterior tibial arteries, left and right dorsalis pedis arteries, dorsal metatarsal arteries, etc.
4. Arterioles and capillaries
5. Large veins: Superior vena cava, Inferior vena cava.
6. Medium and small size veins
7. Venules

Q.76. Enumerate components of endocrine system?

Ans. (Fig. 1.7)

1. Pituitary gland
2. Hypothalamus
3. Pineal gland

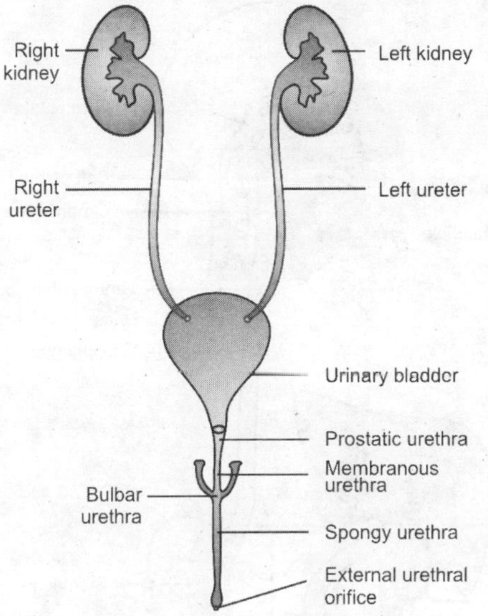

Fig. 1.11: Excretory system

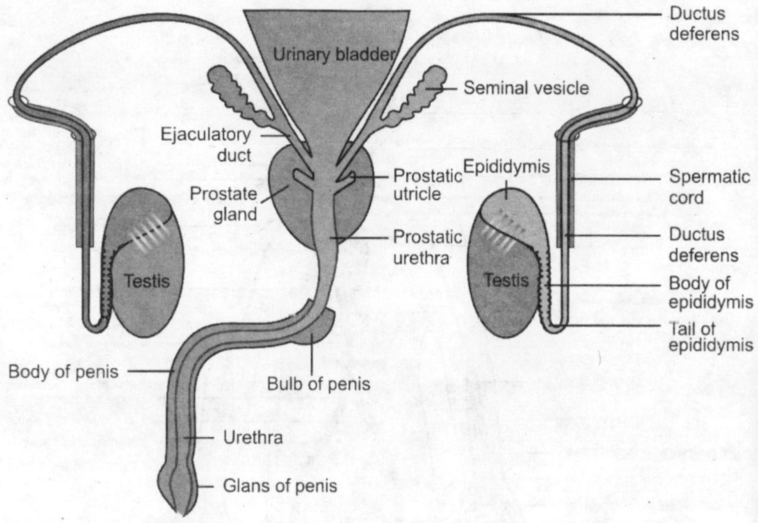

Fig. 1.12: Male reproductive system

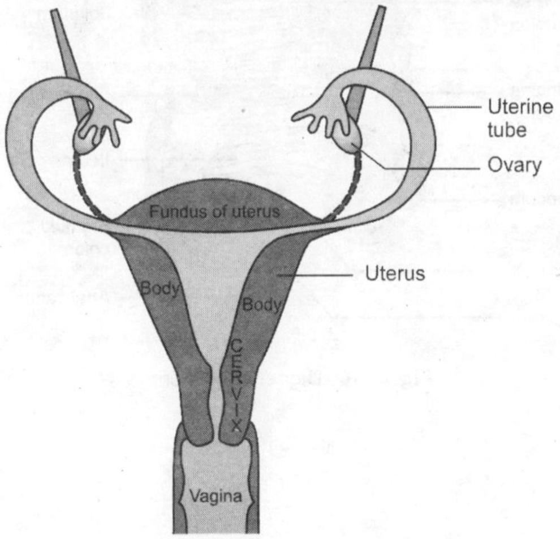

Fig. 1.13: Female reproductive system (Internal genitalia)

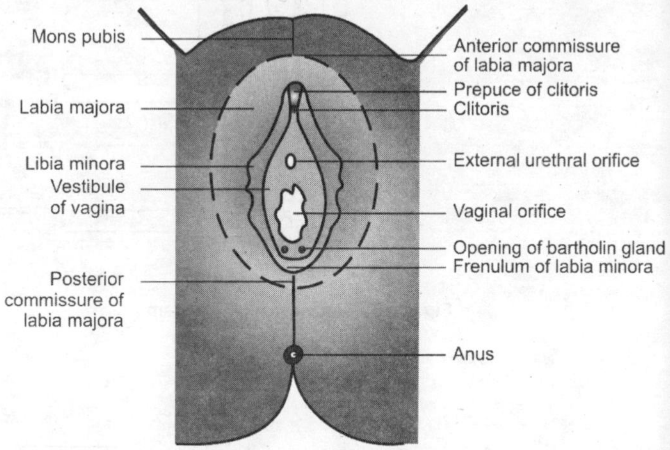

Fig. 1.14: Female reproductive system (External genitalia)

4. Thyroid gland
5. Parathyroid gland
6. Thymus gland
7. Adrenal gland
8. Islets of langerhans
9. Ovary and testis
10. Other organs with endocrine functions are kidneys, mucosa of GIT, skin, placenta (during pregnancy).

Q.77. Name the parts of digestive system?

Ans. (Fig. 1.16)

1. Oral cavity
2. Pharynx
3. Esophagus
4. Stomach
5. Small intestine: Duodenum, jejunum, ileum.
6. Large intestine: Caecum, appendix, ascending colon, transverse colon, descending colon, sigmoid colon, rectum and anal canal.

It is associated with various organs that help in digestion and absorption of food. These are

1. Three pairs of salivary glands: Parotid, submandibular and sublingual glands.
2. Liver and biliary tract
3. Pancreas

Q.78. What is muscular system?

Ans. It consists of muscles and tendons (Fig. 1.17)

Functions of muscular system:

1. Responsible for movement of skeleton and various hollow viscera of the body.
2. Is the site of heat production in body.

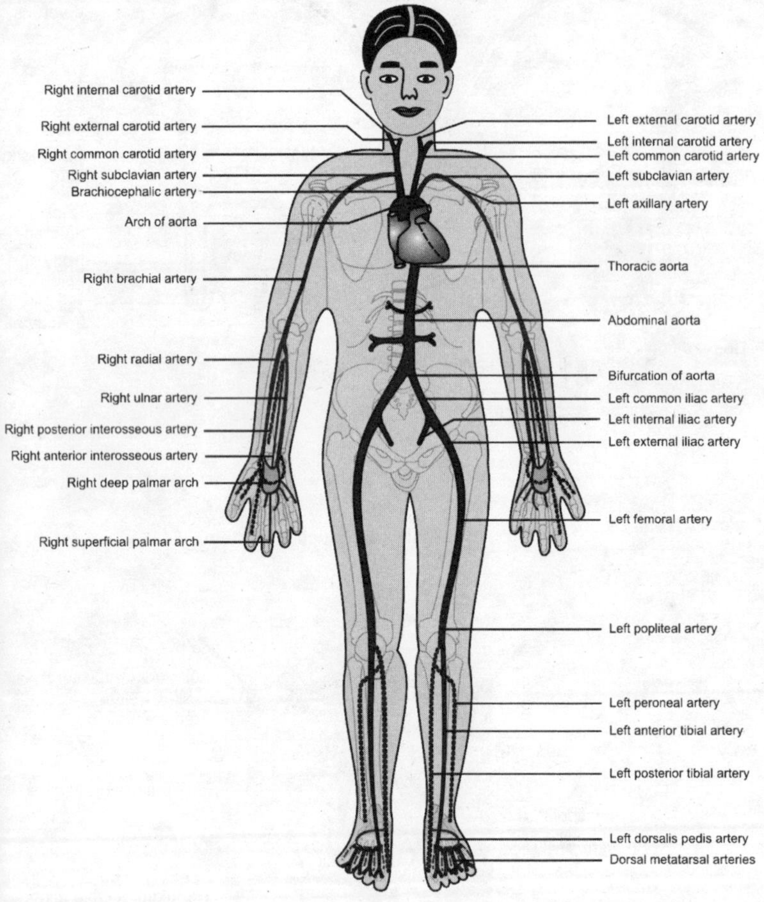

Fig. 1.15: Cardviovascular system

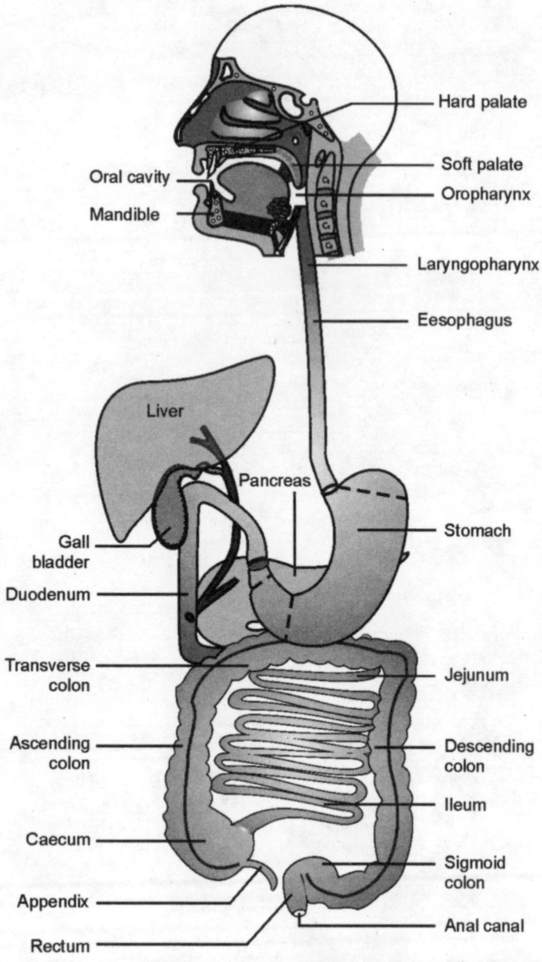

Fig. 1.16: Digestive system

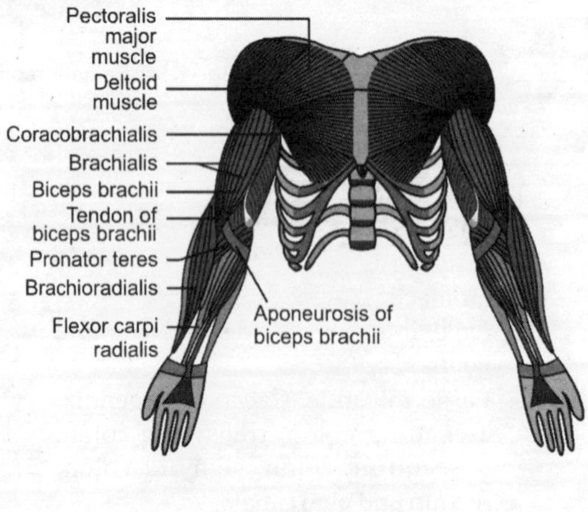

Fig. 1.17: Muscular system

Head and Neck

Q.79. Enumerate bones forming skull?

Ans. Skull is made up of 22 + 6 bones namely (Figs 1.18 to 1.20):

1. Paired bones
   - Temporal
   - Parietal
   - Maxilla
   - Lacrimal
   - Palatine
   - Zygomatic
   - Nasal
   - Inferior concha
2. Unpaired bones
   - Frontal
   - Occipital
   - Sphenoid
   - Ethmoid
   - Vomer
   - Mandible
3. Bones of middle ear cavity
   - Incus
   - Malleus
   - Stapes

Q.80. What is bregma?

Ans. Point at which the coronal and sagittal sutures meet is called bregma (Fig. 1.18).

Q.81. What is Lambda?

Ans. Point at which the sagittal and lambdoid sutures meet is named as lambda (Fig. 1.18).

Q.82. What is pterion?

Ans. It is the region in the anterior part of temporal fossa where 4 bones namely, frontal, parietal, squamo-temporal and greater wing of sphenoid meet to form an H-shaped suture. It is situated 4 cm above the midpoint of the zygomatic arch (Fig. 1.20).

Q.83 What is the clinical significance of pterion?

Ans. Inner aspect of the pterion is related to middle meningeal vessels. In cases of an extradural hematoma due to head injury, where there is injury to middle

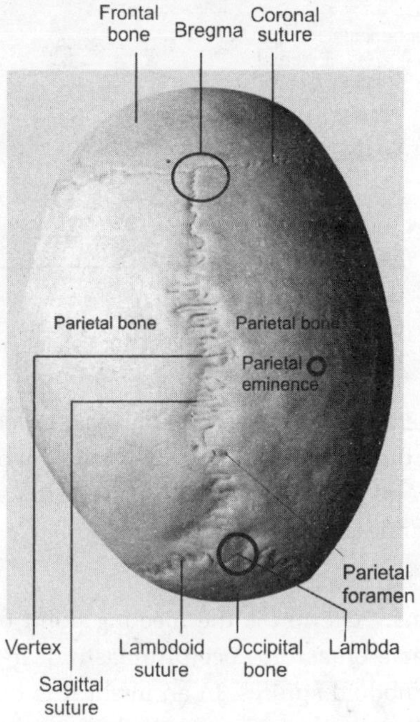

Fig. 1.18: Vertical view of skull

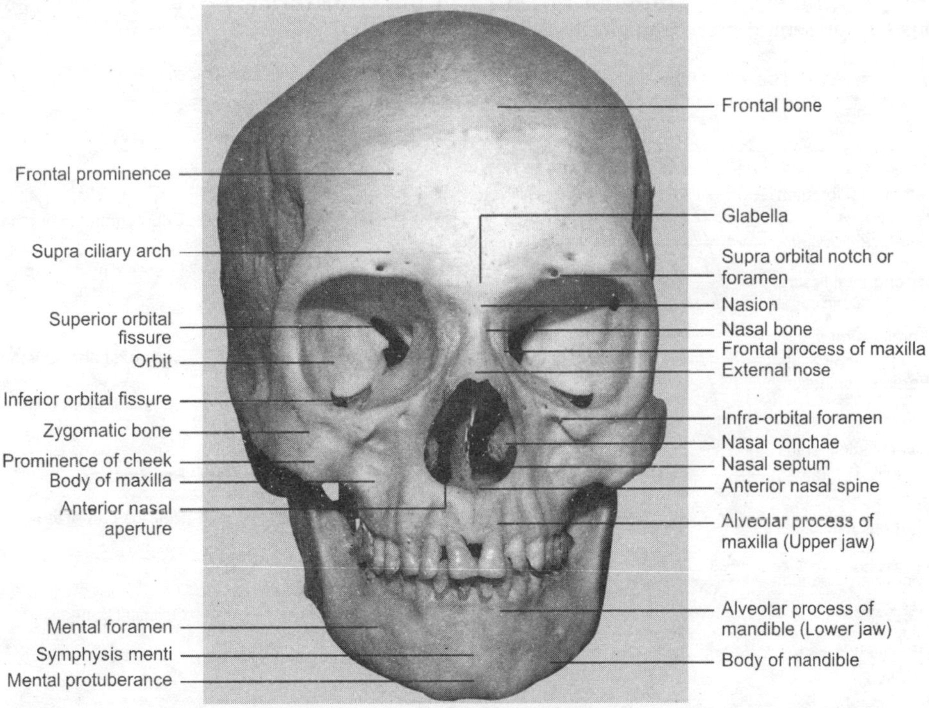

Fig. 1.19: Frontal view of skull

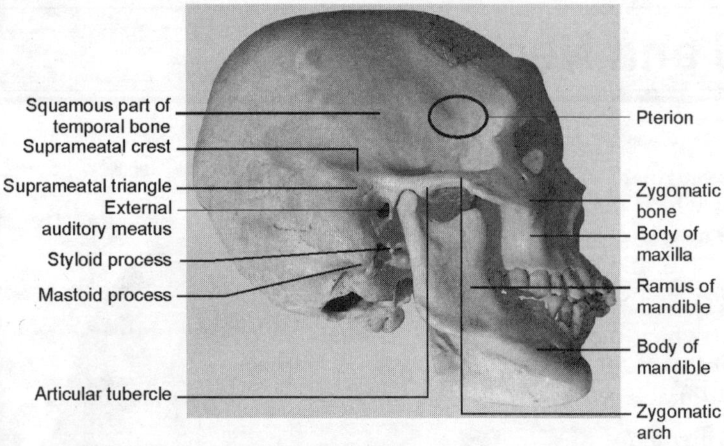

Fig. 1.20: Lateral view of skull

meningeal vessels, a burr hole is drilled in the region of pterion for evacuation of blood to release the pressure. This is thinnest part of upper part of skull.

Q.84. What is asterion?

Ans. Asterion is the meeting point of parietomastoid, occipitomastoid and lambdoid sutures. In an infant it is the site of posterolateral (mastoid) fontanelle.

Q.85. What is anterior fontanelle?

Ans. Anterior fontanelle is a rhomboid shaped membranous gap present at the meeting point of sagittal, coronal and metopic sutures in a new born. It closes by 18 to 24 months of age due to growth of surrounding bones.

Q.86. What is posterior fontanelle?

Ans. Posterior fontanelle is a triangular shaped membranous gap present at junction of sagittal and lamboid sutures in a new born. It closes by 4 months of age due to growth of surrounding bones.

Q.87. Enumerate the structures passing through foramina in the cribriform plate of the ethmoid?

Ans.

1. Olfactory nerves: Surrounded by leptomeninges (pia and arachnoid maters) from olfactory epithelium of the nasal cavity to the olfactory bulb. They are 15-20 in number on each side.
2. Nervi-terminalis

Q.88. What are structures passing through anterior ethmoidal foramen?

Ans.

1. Anterior ethmoidal nerve, branch of nasociliary nerve.
2. Anterior ethmoidal artery, branch of ophthalmic artery.
3. Anterior ethmoidal vein, tributary of ophthalmic vein.

Q.89. What are structures passing through posterior ethmoidal foramen?

Ans. (Fig. 1.21)

1. Posterior ethmoidal nerve, branch of nasociliary nerve.
2. Posterior ethmoidal artery, branch of ophthalmic artery.
3. Posterior ethmoidal vein, tributary of ophthalmic vein

Q.90. What are structures passing through optic foramen?

Ans. (Fig. 1.21)

1. Optic nerve: It passes from the optic disk along with its sheath of meninges, i.e., Duramater, arachnoid mater and piamater.

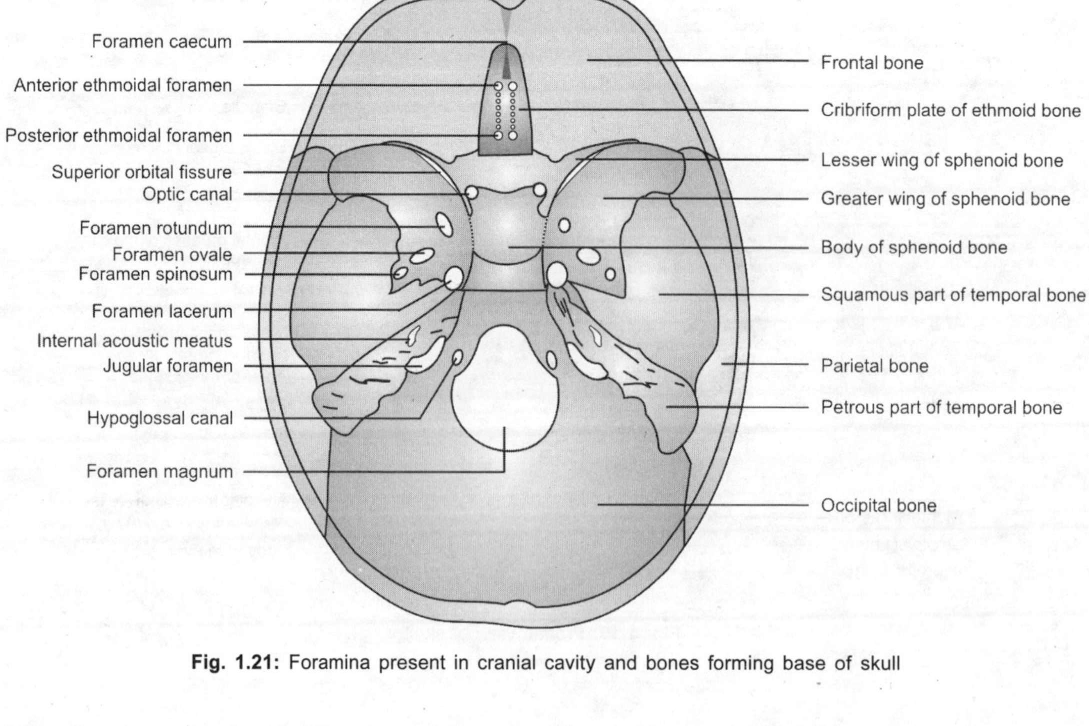

Fig. 1.21: Foramina present in cranial cavity and bones forming base of skull

2. Ophthalmic artery, branch of cerebral part of internal carotid artery. It lies inferolateral to optic nerve.
3. Sympathetic plexus: This plexus consists of post ganglionic sympathetic nerve fibers derived from the superior cervical sympathetic ganglion and it surrounds the ophthalmic artery.

Q.91. What structures pass through superior orbital fissure?

Ans. This fissure is divided into three parts by means of the common tendinous ring of Zinn (Fig. 1.22).

1. Structures passing through the part within the common tendinous ring.
   a. Superior and inferior divisions of oculomotor nerve.
   b. Nasociliary nerve: It lies between the two divisions of oculomotor nerve.
   c. Abducent nerve: It lies posterior to the nasociliary nerve.
   d. Sympathetic root of the ciliary ganglion.
2. Structures passing through the part above the common tendinous ring
   a. Trochlear nerve
   b. Frontal nerve
   c. Lacrimal nerve
   d. Lacrimal artery
   e. Superior ophthalmic vein
   f. Recurrent meningeal branch of lacrimal artery.
3. Structures passing through the part below the common tendinous ring
   a. Inferior ophthalmic vein.

Q.92. What structures pass through foramen rotundum?

Ans. (Figs 1.21 and 1.23)

1. Maxillary nerve, 2nd division of the trigeminal nerve
2. Emissary vein

Q.93. What structures pass through foramen ovale?

Ans. Pnemonic: Male (Figs 1.21 and 1.23)

1. Mandibular nerve, 3rd division of trigeminal nerve.
2. Accessory middle meningeal artery, branch of 1st part of maxillary artery
3. Lesser petrosal nerve
4. Emissary vein, connecting pterygoid venous plexus to the cavernous sinus.

Q.94. Enumerate structures passing through foramen spinosum?

Ans. (Figs 1.21 and 1.23)

1. Middle meningeal artery, branch from 1st part of maxillary artery
2. Nervus spinosus, branch from the undivided trunk of mandibular nerve.
3. Middle meningeal vein

Q.95. Enumerate structures passing through foramen lacerum?

Ans. (Fig. 1.23)

1. Meningeal branch of ascending pharyngeal artery
2. Emissary vein, from cavernous sinus to pharyngeal venous plexus.
3. The anterior part of foramen lacerum lodges the internal carotid artery along with the sympathetic plexus around it.
4. Greater petrosal nerve joins the deep pertrosal nerve to form the nerve of the pterygoid canal or Vidian's nerve.

Q.96. What structures pass through carotid canal?

Ans. (Fig. 1.23)

1. Internal carotid artery.
2. Sympathetic plexus derived from the superior cervical sympathetic ganglion surrounding the artery. This plexus consists of postganglionic fibers.
3. Emissary vein, it connects pharyngeal venous plexus to the cavernous sinus.

Q.97. What structures pass through internal auditory meatus?

Ans.

1. Facial nerve
2. Vestibulo-cochlear nerve
3. Nervus intermedius
4. Internal auditory (labyrinthine) vessels – Internal auditory artery is a branch of basilar artery.

Q.98. Enumerate structures passing through jugular foramen.

Ans. Jugular foramen may be divided into 3 compartments, anterior, middle and posterior

1. Anterior compartment
   a. Inferior petrosal sinus, tributary of internal jugular vein.
2. Middle compartment, from antero-posterior direction
   a. Glossopharyngeal nerve
   b. Vagus nerve
   c. Accessory nerve

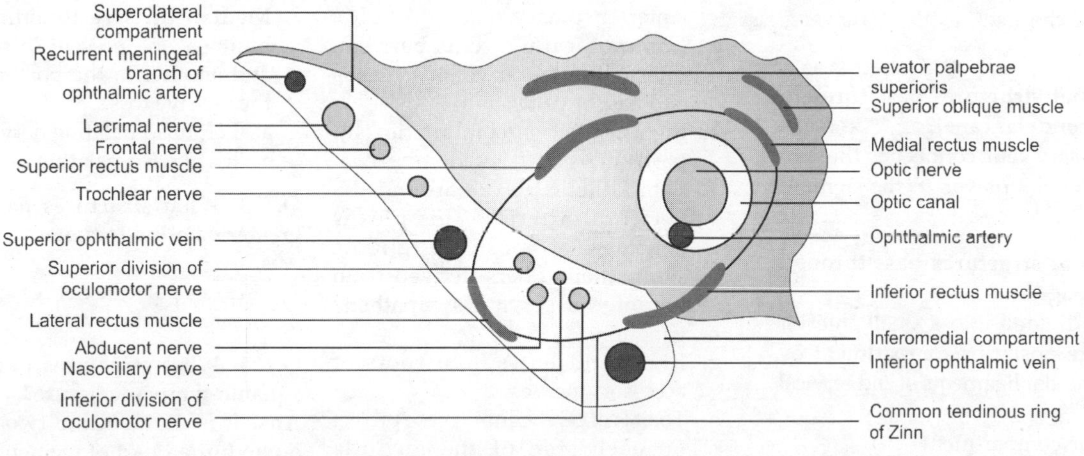

Fig. 1.22: Structures passing through superior orbital fissure

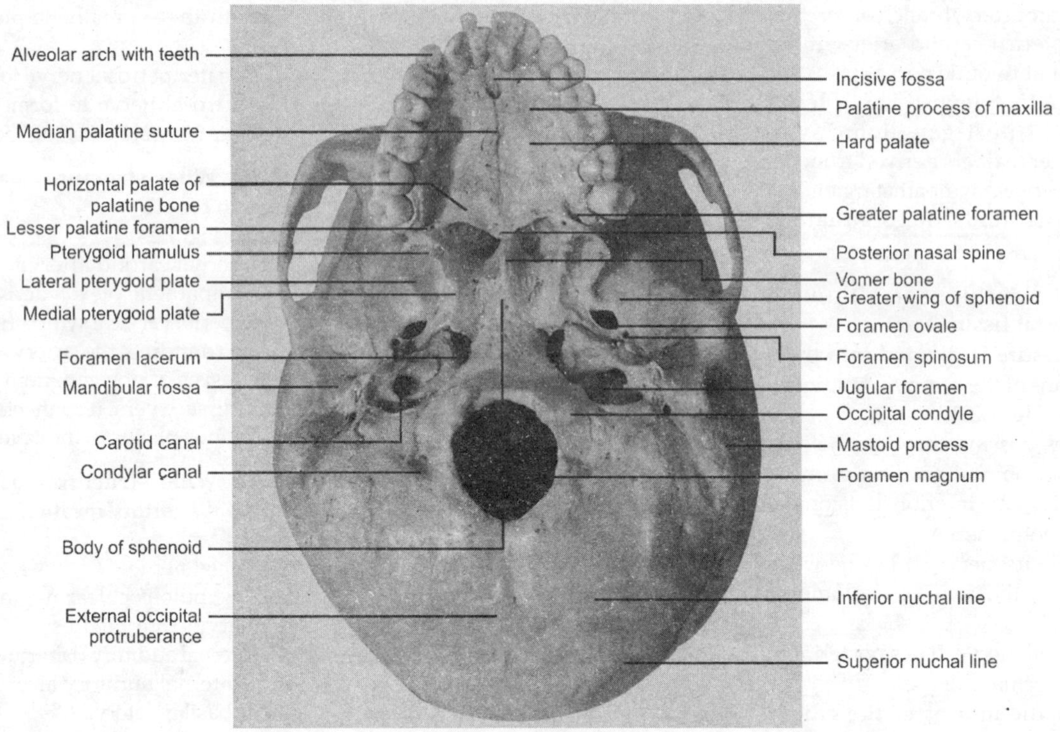

Fig. 1.23: Bones forming base of skull and foramina present

3. Posterior compartment
   a. Sigmoid sinus: It continues as the superior bulb of internal jugular vein.

Q.99. What structures pass through hypoglossal (anterior condylar) canal?

Ans.

1. Hypoglossal nerve
2. Meningeal branch of ascending pharyngeal artery
3. Emissary vein connecting the deep veins of the neck to the transverse sinus.

Q.100. What structures pass through posterior condylar canal?

Ans. Emissary vein, connecting the sub-occipital venous plexus to the sigmoid sinus.

Q.101. What structures pass through foramen magnum?

Ans. It is divided into a small anterior and a large posterior compartment by means of the alar ligaments of 2nd cervical vertebra.

1. Anterior compartment
   a. Apical ligament of dens.
   b. Upper longitudinal band of cruciform ligament.
   c. Membrana tectoria—A continuation of posterior longitudinal ligament of the vertebral bodies.
   d. Process of dens—sometimes.
2. Posterior compartment
   a. Medulla oblongata along with its meninges, i.e. duramater, arachnoid mater and pia mater.
   b. Right and left posterior spinal arteries
   c. Anterior spinal artery
   d. Communicating veins between internal vertebral venous plexus and basilar veins
   e. Right and left vertebral arteries (4th part)
   f. Sympathetic plexus around the vertebral arteries. This plexus consists of post ganglionic sympathetic fibers derived from the inferior cervical sympathetic ganglion.
   g. Right and left spinal roots of accessory nerves
   h. Tonsils of cerebellum: These project on each side of the medulla oblongata.

Q.102. What structures pass through incisive foramina?

Ans.

1. **Lateral incisive foramina:** Two in number, right and left, are present in the lateral wall of the incisive fossa. Each leads into the floor of the nasal cavity through the incisive canal and transmits:
   a. Greater palatine vessels
   b. Naso-palatine nerve, only when the median foramina are absent.
2. **Median incisive foramina:** Two in number, one present in the anterior and another in the posterior wall of the incisive fossa.
   a. Left naso-palatine nerve
   b. Right naso-palatine nerve

Q.103. What structures pass through greater palatine foramen?

Ans.

1. Greater palatine nerves
2. Greater palatine vessels

Q.104. What structures pass through squamo-tympanic fissure?

Ans. It is divided into two parts by a down turned part of tegmen tympani, a part of petrous temporal bone

1. Petro-tympanic fissure
   a. Chorda tympani nerve, branch of facial nerve.
   b. Anterior tympanic artery, branch of 1st part of the maxillary artery
   c. Anterior ligament of the malleus
2. Petro-squamous fissure: No structure passes through it.

Q.105. What structures pass through palatovaginal canal?

Ans.

1. Pharyngeal nerve, branch from pterygopalatine ganglion.
2. Pharyngeal artery, branch of 3rd part of maxillary artery.

Q.106. What structures pass through vomero-vaginal canal?

Ans.

1. Pharyngeal nerve
2. Pharyngeal artery

Q.107. What structures pass through pterygoid canal?

Ans.

1. Nerve of pterygoid canal (Vidian's nerve)
2. Vessels of the pterygoid canal

Q.108. What structures pass through tympanic canaliculus?

Ans. It is located on a bony crest present between the carotid canal and jugular fossa. It provides passage to the tympanic branch of glossopharyngeal nerve (Jacobson's nerve).

Q.109. What structures pass through mastoid canaliculus (Arnold's canal)?

Ans. It is present in the lateral wall of jugular fossa. It provides passage to auricular branch of vagus nerve (Alderman's nerve/Arnold's nerve).

Q.110. What structures pass through stylomastoid foramen?

Ans.

1. 7th cranial (facial nerve)
2. Stylomastoid artery: A branch of posterior auricular artery.

Q.111. What structures pass through zygomatico-temporal foramen?

Ans.

1. Zygomatico-temporal nerve
2. Zygomatico-temporal artery

Q.112. What structures pass through pterygo-maxillary fissure?

Ans.

1. 3rd part of the maxillary artery.
2. Maxillary nerve, 2nd division of the trigeminal nerve.

Q.113. What structures pass through inferior orbital fissure?

Ans.

1. Maxillary nerve
2. Infraorbital vessels
3. Zygomatic nerve
4. Vein connecting inferior ophthalmic vein with pterygoid venous plexus

Q.114. What structures pass through spheno-palatine foramen?

Ans.

1. Nasopalatine nerve
2. Sphenopalatine vessels

Q.115. What structures pass through greater palatine canal?

Ans.

1. Anterior, middle and posterior palatine nerves
2. Greater palatine vessels
3. Lesser palatine vessels

Q.116. What structures pass through supraorbital foramen?

Ans.

1. Supraorbital nerve: A branch of frontal nerve which in turn is a branch of ophthalmic division of trigeminal cranial nerve.
2. Frontal diploic vein

Q.117. What structures pass through infraorbital foramen?

Ans.

1. Infraorbital nerve: Continuation of maxillary nerve.
2. Infraorbital artery: Branch of maxillary artery
3. Infraorbital vein

Q.118. What structures pass through mandibular foramen?

Ans.

1. Inferior alveolar nerve, branch of the posterior division the mandibular nerve.
2. Inferior alveolar artery, branch of 1st part of maxillary artery
3. Inferior alveolar vein

Q.119. What structures pass through mental foramen?

Ans.

1. Mental nerve, branch of inferior alveolar nerve.
2. Mental artery, branch of inferior alveolar artery.
3. Inferior alveolar vein.

Q.120. Name the nerves related to mandible?

Ans. Nerves related to the mandible are (Fig. 1.24)

1. **Lingual nerve:** It runs on the inner surface of the body close to the medial side of the root of the third molar tooth.
2. **Inferior alveolar nerve:** Enters the mandibular foramen and passes through mandibular canal.

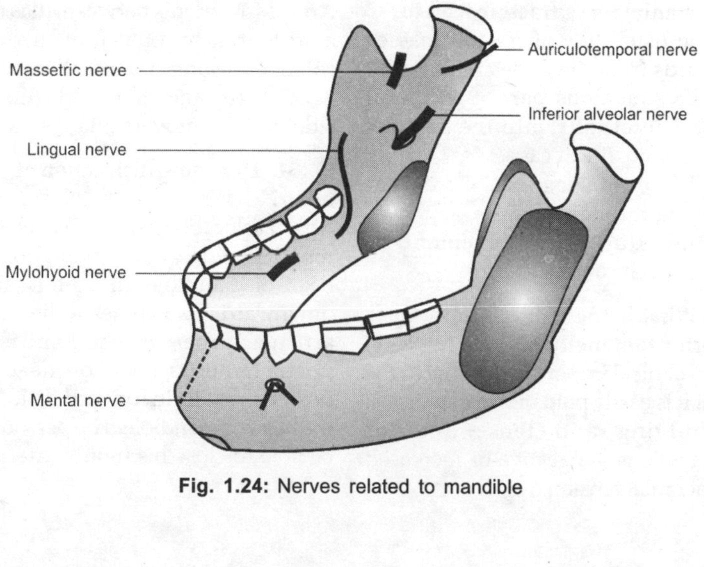

Fig. 1.24: Nerves related to mandible

ANATOMY

3. **Mylohyoid nerve**: Runs in the mylohyoid groove.
4. **Mental nerve:** It comes out of the mental foramen.
5. **Nerve to masseter:** Passes over the mandibular notch.
6. **Auriculo-temporal nerve:** It winds around the medial surface of neck of the condylar process.

Q.121. What is suprameatal triangle?

Ans. It is also known as triangle of McEven. It is a triangular depression present posterosuperior to external auditory meatus. It is bounded by

1. Supramastoid crest, superiorly.
2. Posterosuperior margin of external acoustic meatus, anteriorly.
3. A vertical tangent to the posterior margin of the meatus, posteriorly.

The mastoid antrum lies 12 mm deep to this triangle in adults.

Q.122. What is the clinical importance of suprameatal triangle?

Ans. Severe mastoiditis, needing surgical intervention, is treated by approaching the mastoid antrum via the suprameatal triangle. Careful anatomical delineation is important as it is related to the facial nerve posteriorly and the sigmoid sinus anteriorly.

Q.123. What can fracture of anterior cranial fossa lead to?

Ans. A fracture involving the cribriform plate of ethmoid can cause bleeding and/or drainage of cerebrospinal fluid (CSF) from the nose. Leaking of CSF is known as rhinorrhea.

Q.124. What can head injury, causing middle cranial fossa fracture lead to?

Ans. The usual line of fracture passes downwards from the parietal tuberosity along the squamous part of temporal bone and internally into the petrous temporal bone. It can cause:

1. Bleeding or drainage of CSF from ear
2. Bleeding through nose
3. Vertigo due to involvement of semicircular canals.

Q.125. What is the clinical importance of anterior fontanelle?

Ans. Its clinical importance is due to the fact that it is easily palpated in newborns.

1. A bulging and tense anterior fontanelle is suggestive of increased intracranial tension.
2. A depressed fontanelle is a sign of dehydration in newborn.
3. The superior sagittal sinus lies below this fontanelle.
4. During labor the position of anterior fontanelle helps to identify the position of fetal head in the maternal pelvis.

Q.126. What is carotid tubercle?

Ans. The anterior tubercle of the transverse process of sixth cervical vertebra is large and called the carotid tubercle because common carotid artery can be compressed and felt against it.

Q.127. What is hangman's fracture?

Ans. The death in execution by hanging is due to fracture of odontoid process of axis vertebra with subsequent posterior dislocation of atlas vertebra which compresses the medulla resulting in death.

Q.128. What is the applied importance of joints of Luschka?

Ans. Luschka's joints are very common sites of osteophyte formation. Since cervical nerve roots lie posterolateral to these joints, the osteophytes may produce symptoms due to cervical nerve compression. The osteophytes may also intrude on the foramina transversaria transmitting vertebral artery. This may cause distortion of the artery which produces vertebro-basilar insufficiency.

Q.129. What is 'yes' movement?

Ans. Movements between the atlas and the skull at atlanto occipital joints are flexion and extension, i.e. 'nodding' or 'yes' movements.

Q.130. What is 'no' movement?

Ans. Movements between atlas and axis at the atlanto-axial joint are mainly rotation around a vertical axis, dens of axis, i.e. 'turning the head from side to side' or 'No' movements.

Q.131. How does dislocation of TM joint occur?

Ans. Dislocation usually occurs when the mouth is widely open. In this position the head of mandible glides forwards and downwards and comes to lie below the articular tubercle. The joint is highly unstable and a blow on head in this position results in forward dislocation of the head of mandible. The person will not be able to close his mouth after such an injury.

Q.132. What are layers of scalp?

Ans. The soft tissues of the scalp are arranged in five layers:

S – Skin
C – Connective tissue
A – Aponeurosis
L – Loose areolar tissue
P – Periosteum

Q.133. Which is the dangerous layer of scalp?

Ans. Loose areolar tissue layer is the dangerous layer of scalp.

Q.134. What is caput?

Ans. Caput is the collection of fluid in the loose aerolar tissue of scalp due to forces of labor. The swelling due to caput is generally diffuse and more on the dependant areas instead of a particular bone and also crosses the midline as it is not limited to sutures.

Q.135. Why do scalp wounds bleed profusely?

Ans. The neurovascular bundle of scalp lies in the tough connective tissue layer of scalp. In case of injury to the scalp, this tough connective tissue prevents the retraction of blood vessels. Therefore, scalp wounds bleed profusely.

Q.136. Why does black eye occur in cases of head injuries?

Ans. Head injury resulting in soft tissue damage can cause collection of blood in the loose subaponeurotic layer of scalp which is continuous with the upper eye lid. The blood easily tracks down anteriorly over the eyelids leading to discoloration of the eyelids known as black eye. The spread of this collection is limited posteriorly and laterally due to attachment of the aponeurosis to the supranuchal lines and zygomatic arches at these points.

Q.137. What is cephalhematoma? How does it differ from a fluid collection in the loose areolar tissue of the scalp?

Ans. Cephalhematoma is the collection of blood below the periosteal layer of scalp due to an injury. The swelling due to the hematoma is localized over the particular bone involved as the periosteum is adherent to the underlying bone at the sutures which limits its spread. In cases of collection of fluid or blood in the loose aerolar tissue, e.g. caput formation in a newborn (due to forces of labor), the swelling is generally diffuse and more on the dependant areas instead of a particular bone. Caput also crosses the midline as it is not limited by sutures.

Q.138. Which is the smiling muscle of face?

Ans. Zygomaticus major and minor.

Q.139. Which muscle is involved in expression of surprise?

Ans. Frontalis and Procerus.

Q.140. Which muscle is involved in expression of frowning?

Ans. Corrugator supercilli.

Q.141. Which muscle is involved in expression of anger?

Ans. Dilator naris and depressor septi

Q.142. Which muscle is involved in expression of laughing and smiling?

Ans. Zygomaticus major

Q.143. Which muscle is involved in expression of sadness?

Ans. Depressor anguli oris

Q.144. Which muscle is involved in expression of sorrow and grief?

Ans.

1. Levator labii superioris
2. Levator anguli oris
3. Zygomaticus minor

Q.145. Which muscle is involved in expression of grinning?

Ans. Risorius.

Q.146. Which muscle is involved in expression of disdain or doubt?

Ans. Mentalis.

Q.147. Which muscle is involved in expression of whistling?

Ans. Buccinator.

Q.148. What is dangerous area of face?

Ans. Dangerous area of face comprises of lower part of nose, upper lip and the adjoining cheek. This area is drained by facial vein. The facial vein communicates with the cavernous sinus via ophthalmic veins and pterygoid plexus of veins. The facial vein does not contain valves and it rests directly on the muscles of facial expressions. Contraction of these muscles aid the retrograde spread of any infective embolus from an infected part in the area mentioned above. It can thus reach the cavernous sinus and cause thrombosis which can be fatal.

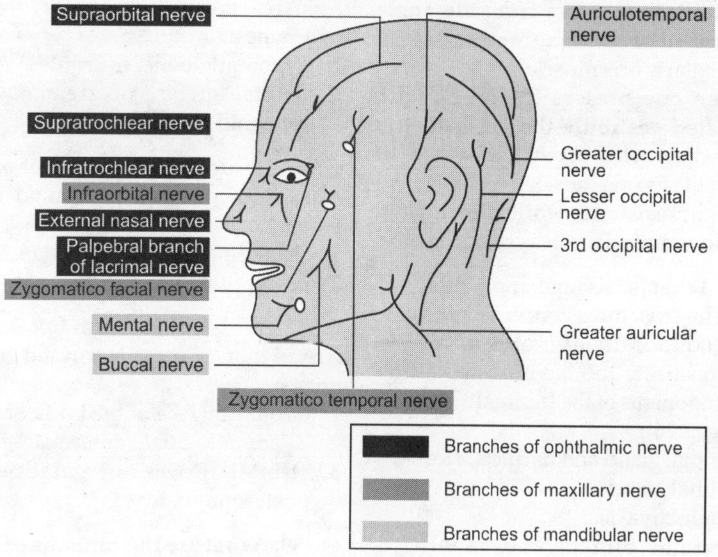

Fig. 1.25: Sensory supply of face

Q.149. What is the sensory supply of face?

Ans. The face receives its sensory innervation from following two sources (Fig. 1.25):

1. *Trigeminal nerve:* The three divisions of trigeminal nerve supply almost the entire skin of face except an area over the angle of mandible. The various branches supplying face are:
   a. From ophthalmic division
      - Lacrimal nerve
      - Supraorbital nerve
      - Supratrochlear nerve
      - Infratrochlear nerve
      - External nasal nerve
   b. From maxillary division
      - Infraorbital nerve
      - Zygomatico-facial nerve
      - Zygomatico-temporal nerve
   c. From mandibular division
      - Mental branch
      - Buccal branch
      - Auriculotemporal nerve
2. *Great auricular nerve (C_2):* This branch of cervical plexus supplies the area of skin over the angle of mandible.

Q.150. What is motor supply of face?

Ans. Nerve supply to the muscles of the face is derived from the facial nerve and its 5 branches:

1. Temporal
2. Zygomatic
3. Buccal
4. Marginal mandibular
5. Cervical

Q.151. What is Bell's palsy?

Ans. Bell's palsy is a lower motor neuron type of palsy of the facial nerve due to compression of the nerve in the facial canal near stylomastoid foramen. The exact etiology is not known but it is probably due to a viral infection. Facial muscles of the same side are paralysed.

Q.152. What are the features of Bell's Palsy?

Ans.

1. **Facial asymmetry:** Due to unopposed action of muscles of the normal side. There is deviation of angle of mouth to the opposite side.
2. **Loss of wrinkles on forehead:** Due to paralysis of fronto-occipitalis muscle.
3. **Widening of palpebral fissure and inability to close the eye:** Due to paralysis of orbicularis oculi muscle.
4. **Inability of angle of mouth to move upwards and laterally during laughing:** Due to paralysis of zygomaticus major muscle.
5. **Loss of naso-labial furrow:** It is due to paralysis of levator labii superioris alaeque nasi muscle.
6. **Accumulation of food into the vestibule of mouth:** Due to paralysis of buccinator muscle.

7. **Dribbling of saliva from the angle of mouth:** Due to paralysis of orbicularis oris muscle.
8. **When one presses the cheek with inflated vestibule the air leaks out between the lips:** Paralysis of orbicularis oris muscle.
9. **Loss of resistance while blowing out air in mouth:** Paralysis of buccinator.

Q.153. What is lacrimal apparatus?
Ans. The structures concerned with the production and drainage of lacrimal (tear) fluid constitute the lacrimal apparatus. The components of the lacrimal apparatus are (Fig. 1.26):
1. Lacrimal gland and its ducts, accessory lacrimal glands
2. Conjunctival sac
3. Lacrimal puncta and canaliculi, common canaliculus
4. Lacrimal sac
5. Nasolacrimal duct

Q.154. Name the glands present in eye lid?
Ans. Zies glands, Moll's glands and Meibomian or tarsal glands.

Q.155. Which bones form medial wall of orbit?
Ans. Medial wall of orbit is formed by four bones. They are, from before backwards:
1. Frontal process of maxilla
2. Lacrimal bone
3. Orbital plate of ethmoid
4. Body of sphenoid

Q.156. Which bones form lateral wall of orbit?
Ans. Lateral wall of orbit is formed by two bones:
1. Zygomatic bone, in front
2. Orbital surface of greater wing of sphenoid, behind

Q.157. Which bones form roof of orbit?
Ans. Roof of orbit is formed by two bones:
1. Orbital plate of frontal bone, in front
2. Lesser wing of sphenoid, behind

Q.158. Which bones form floor of orbit?
Ans. Floor of orbit is formed by three bones:
1. Orbital surface of the body of maxilla
2. Zygomatic bone, anterolaterally
3. Orbital process of palatine bone, posteromedially

Q.159. What are the contents of orbit?
Ans. Contents of orbit are:
1. Eyeball
2. Muscles of orbit
3. Fascia bulbi
4. Nerves:
   a. Optic nerve
   b. 3rd, 4th and 6th cranial nerves
   c. Ophthalmic nerve
5. Ophthalmic artery
6. Superior and inferior ophthalmic veins
7. Lacrimal gland
8. Orbital fat

Q.160. What are layers of eye ball?
Ans. The eyeball consists of three concentric coats:
1. An outer fibrous coat, consisting of sclera and cornea
2. A middle vascular coat, consisting of choroid, ciliary body and iris
3. An inner nervous coat, consisting of retina

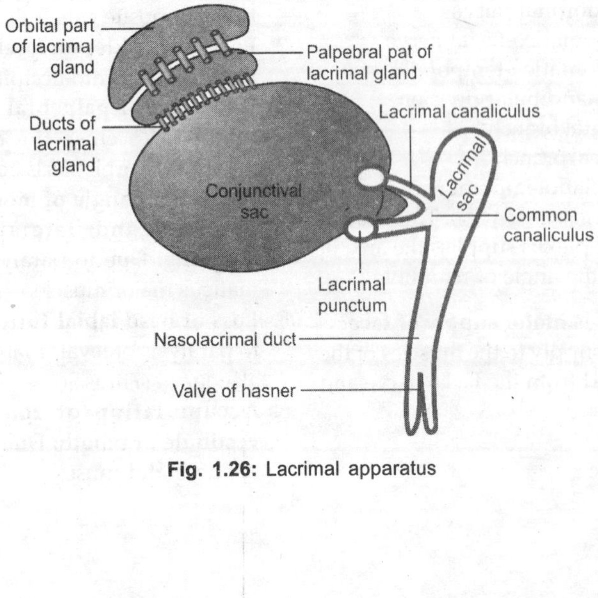

Fig. 1.26: Lacrimal apparatus

Q.161. What is macula?
Ans. It is a pale yellowish area seen near the posterior pole of fundus with ophthalmoscope. It is approximately 5 mm in diameter. A small pit in its center is called the fovea centralis. This is the point where light is normally focused. Fovea is that portion of retina which has the maximum concentration of cones. Hence, it is the site of greatest visual acuity i.e. the ability to see fine images.

Q.162. What is visual pathway or optic pathway?
Ans. The retina is the photoreceptive layer of the eye and impulses generated in rods and cones of retina are finally transmitted along the axons of ganglion cells of retina which converge to the optic disk and exit the eyeball as optic nerve.
1. The impulses course through optic nerve, optic chiasma and optic tract to relay in lateral geniculate body of corresponding side.
2. The fibers originating from nasal halves of the retina cross to opposite side at the chiasma. Hence each optic tract consists of fibers from temporal region of retina of ipsilateral side and nasal region of retina of contra-lateral side.
3. The fibers from nuclei of lateral geniculate body extend to the visual cortex in the medial aspect of occipital lobe via the optic radiation.

Q.163. What is pupillary light reflex?
Ans. Pupillary light reflex is defined as constriction of the pupil of the eye when it is exposed to bright illumination.

Q.164. What is the pathway of pupillary light reflex?
Ans. The path of nerve impulses causing this reflex is as follows:
1. On stimulation with bright light the nerve impulses pass through ganglion cells of retina, optic, nerve, optic chiasma and optic tract to pretectal nucleus of mid brain.
2. Fibers of secondary neurons from pretectal nuclei then convey impulses to the Edinger-Westphal nuclei bilaterally.
3. Preganglionic fibers from Edinger-Wesphal nuclei carry impulses to ciliary ganglia via oculomotor nerve.

4. Postganglionic fibers from ciliary ganglion on each side travel along short ciliary nerves to supply sphincter pupillae muscle which contracts in response.

Q.165. What are direct and indirect light reflexes?

Ans. When one eye exposed to a beam of light the pupil of both eyes constrict together and equally. Constriction of pupil which is exposed to beam of light is called direct light reflex while simultaneous constriction of pupil of opposite eye is called consensual or indirect light reflex.

Q.166. What is near vision reflex?

Ans. In order to view near objects the eyes respond by:

1. Convergence of eyes
2. Contraction of ciliary muscles leading to change in shape of anterior surface of lens, accommodation reflex.
3. Constriction of pupils to increase depth of focus.

Q.167. What is near vision pathway?

Ans.

1. Afferent path is along optic nerves, optic chiasma, optic tracts, lateral geniculate bodies, optic radiation to the visual areas in cerebral cortex. Then impulses are transmitted to pretectal region and Edinger-Westphal and motor nuclei of oculomotor nerve via superior longitudinal fasciculus, frontal eye field and internal capsule.
2. Efferent path consisting parasympathetic fibers arises from Edinger-Westphal nucleus and travel along oculomotor nerve to relay in ciliary ganglion. Post ganglionic fibers supply ciliary muscle and sphincter pupillae via short ciliary nerves.
3. Efferent fibers from oculomotor nerve supply medial rectus muscle of eyeball.

Q.168. What is stye?

Ans. Stye is an acute suppurative inflammation of a Zies gland. The pus points near the base of the cilia. Epilation of the concerned eyelash helps to drain the pus.

Q.169. What is chalazion?

Ans. Chalazion (internal stye) is the inflammation of a tarsal (meibomian) gland. The swelling points on the inner aspect of the eyelid.

Q.170. What is dacrgocystitis?

Ans. Inflammation of lacrimal sac is called dacryocystitis. It hampers the drainage of lacrimal fluid into the nose. This causes over flow of the lacrimal fluid from the conjunctival sac on to the face, a condition called **epiphora**.

Q.171. What happens in case of unilateral ocular muscle paralysis?

Ans. Unilateral paralysis of an individual extra ocular muscle, due to involvement of the corresponding nerve, produces strabismus or squint and may result in diplopia (double vision). Diplopia occurs because the light from an object is not focussed on identical areas of both retinae. The real image falls on the macula of the unaffected eye while the false image falls on some peripheral part of the retina in the paralysed eye leading to diplopia.

Q.172. What is the clinical importance of levator palpebrae superioris?

Ans. Paralysis of levator palpebrae superioris leads to ptosis, i.e. drooping of upper eyelid. This can be due to either, involvement of oculomotor nerve or of the cervical sympathetic chain (as in Horner's syndrome).

Q.173. What is the clinical importance of central artery of retina?

Ans. The central artery of retina is an end artery and obstruction of this artery by an embolism or pressure results in sudden total blindness.

Q.174. What is arcus senilis?

Ans. Due to ageing there is fatty degeneration along the periphery of the cornea. This becomes visible as a white ring in old people and is known as arcus senilis.

Q.175. What is retinal detachment?

Ans. In retinal detachment there is separation of the two layers of retina. Retinal pigment epithelium separates from the neurosensory layer of retina.

Q.176. What is papilledema?

Ans. Normal optic disk appears on ophthalmoscopy as a cup shaped area, paler than the surrounding area, i.e. the fundus. The edges of the cup are sharp and well-defined. In patients with raised intracranial pressure the optic disk is congested and the cup gets obscured and the disk margin is blurred. This is known as papilledema. The intracranial pressure gets transmitted to the disk via the meningeal coverings which continue over the optic nerve. The raised pressure also compresses the central retinal artery which lies in the subarachnoid space around the optic nerve.

Q.177. What is glaucoma?

Ans. An abnormal increase in intraocular pressure leads to the condition called glaucoma. This occurs due to a block in the circulation and drainage of the aqueous humor. In acute conditions there is severe pain due to pressure on the highly sensitive cornea. Glaucoma results in pressure necrosis of the retina and eventually can cause blindness.

Q.178. What is accommodation?

Ans. The change in focal length of the lens of the eye when it focuses on a nearby object is called accommodation.

This occurs by the contraction of ciliary muscles and enables us to see both the far and near objects with the same lens.

Q.179. What is cataract?

Ans. Opacification of the lens is known as cataract. The most common cause is senile cataract.

Q.180. What is presbiopia?

Ans. It is the gradual loss of power of accommodation of the lens due to changes secondary to ageing as mentioned above. The lens plays an important role in accomodation and as it hardens with age it looses its flexibility.

Q.181. What is pachymeninx?

Ans. The dura mater is also called pachymeninx.

Q.182. What are leptomeninges?

Ans. The arachnoid and piamater are together known as leptomeninges.

Q.183. Enumerate the folds of duramater covering brain?

Ans. Folds of duramater:

1. Falx cerebri
2. Tentorium cerebrai
3. Falx cerebelli
4. Diaphragma sellae

Q.184. What is extradural hematoma?

Ans. It is the collection of blood between the endosteal layer of duramater and the bone of the skull. It generally occurs following head injury. The commonest vessel involved is the middle meningeal vein followed by middle meningeal artery. The blood gradually collects and strips off the endosteal layer from the skull. The patient may present initially with loss of consciousness for a short duration followed by a lucid interval of normal consciousness. As the intracranial pressure gradually increases the patient again presnts with confusion, drowsiness, paralysis and unconsciousness. Hematoma following injury to anterior branch of middle meningeal artery causes pressure on the motor area of the brain giving rise to hemiplegia of the opposite side. Surgical drainage of hematoma is done by burring a hole through the pterion.

Q.185. What is subdural hematoma?

Ans. It is the collection of blood between the meningeal layer of duramater and the arachnoid mater. It occurs following head injury with damage to superficial cerebral veins.

Q.186. What can be the consequences of a fracture of base of skull?

Ans. If the internal carotid artery is ruptured in a fracture of base of skull, an arterio-venous communication may be established between the artery and cavernous sinus.

The patient presents with following features

1. Pulsating exophthalmos.
2. A loud bruit (loud systolic murmur) that is easily heard over the eye.
3. Ophthalmoplegia due to an increase in the venous pressure of the cavernous sinus which compresses upon the 3rd and 4th cranial nerves.
4. Marked orbital and conjunctival edema because the venous pressure of the cavernous sinus is raised to the arterial pressure.

Q.187. Enumerate the dural venous sinuses?

Ans. Dural venous sinuses – They are classified as 7 paired and 7 unpaired sinuses (Fig. 1.27).

Unpaired sinuses are:

1. Superior sagittal sinus
2. Inferior sagittal sinus
3. Straight sinus
4. Occipital sinus

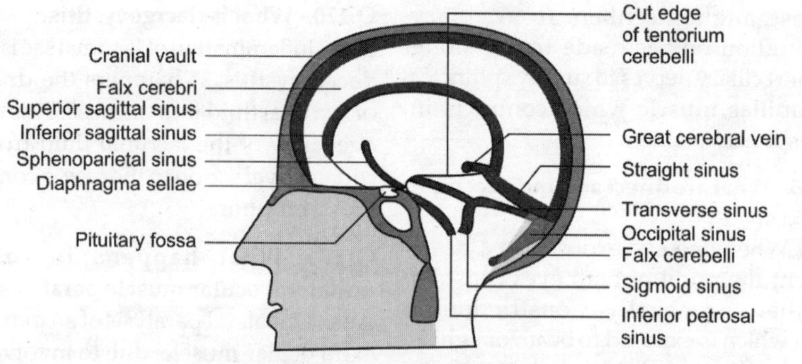

Fig. 1.27: Dural venous sinuses

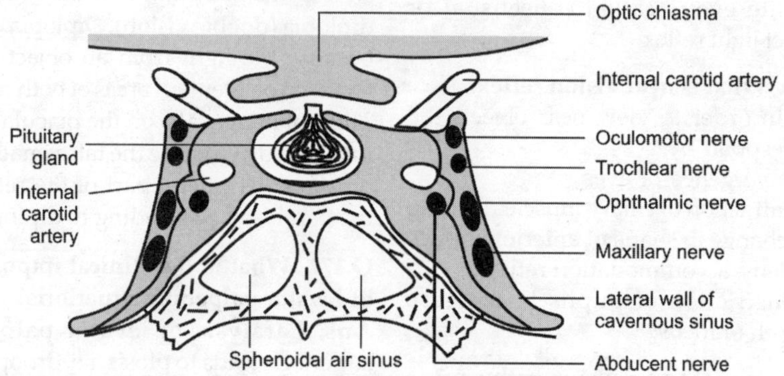

Fig. 1.28: Cavernous sinus

5. Anterior intercavernous sinus
6. Posterior intercavernous sinus
7. Basilar venous plexus (sinus)

Paired sinuses are:

1. Cavernous sinus
2. Superior petrosal sinus
3. Inferior petrosal sinus
4. Transverse sinus
5. Sigmoid sinus
6. Spheno-parietal sinus
7. Petro-squamous sinus

Q.188. What are the characteristic features of dural venous sinuses?

Ans. Characteristic features of the intracranial dural venous sinuses are:

1. The sinuses are present between the two layers of duramater.
2. They are lined by endothelium only, muscular coat is absent.
3. They are valveless.
4. They receive venous blood and CSF.
5. They receive valveless emissary veins which regulate the intracranial blood flow and maintain equilibrium of venous pressure within and outside the skull.

Q.189. What structures are passing through lateral wall of cavernous sinus?

Ans. They are (Fig. 1.28):

1. Oculomotor nerve
2. Trochlear nerve
3. Ophthalmic nerve
4. Maxillary nerve

Q.190. What structures are passing through cavernous sinus?

Ans. They are:

1. Internal carotid artery
2. Abducent nerve

Q.191. Enumerte the tributaries of cavernous sinus?

Ans. Tributaries of cavernous sinus are:

1. From orbit
   a. Superior ophthalmic vein
   b. Inferior ophthalmic vein
   c. Central vein of retina (sometimes)
2. From meninges
   a. Sphenoparietal sinus
   b. Anterior (frontal) trunk of middle meningeal vein
3. From brain
   a. Superior middle cerebral vein
   b. Inferior cerebral veins (only few).

Q.192. What is cavernous sinus thrombosis?

Ans. Thrombosis of cavernous sinus has a varied etiology due to its numerous communications. The commonest cause of thrombosis is due to passage of septic emboli from an infection in the dangerous area of the face through facial plexus of veins to the deep facial vein then to the pterygoid venous plexus and finally via emissary vein into the sinus.

Q.193. What are featurs of cavernous sinus thrombosis

Ans. Features of cavernous sinus thrombosis:

1. Severe pain in the eye and forehead, due to involvement of ophthalmic nerve.
2. Ophthalmoplegia, paralysis of extra ocular muscles due to involvement of 3rd, 4th and 6th cranial nerves.
3. Marked edema of eyelids with exophthalmos, due to congestion of orbital veins following obstruction of ophthalmic veins.

Q.194. What is the clinical importance of sigmoid sinus?

Ans. The sigmoid sinus is separated from the mastoid antrum and mastoid air cells by a thin plate of bone only. Thrombosis of the sigmoid sinus therefore can occur secondary to an infection of the middle ear or mastoid process. It is for the same reason that utmost care should be taken not to expose the sigmoid sinus during operations on the mastoid process.

Q.195. What are emissary veins?

Ans. Emissary veins are channels between intracranial venous sinuses and the extracranial veins. They pass along the various foramina of the skull.

Their clinical significance lies in the fact that they can aid the spread of extra cranial infections into the cranial cavity.

Q.196. Eumerate important emissary veins?

Ans.

1. **Mastoid emissary veins:** It connects sigmoid sinus with posterior auricular or occipital vein via the mastoid foramen.
2. **Parietal emissary vein:** It connects superior sagittal sinus with veins of scalp via parietal foramen.
3. **Venous plexus in hypoglossal canal:** It connects sigmoid sinus with internal jugular vein.
4. **Condylar emissary vein:** It connects sigmoid sinus to the veins in the suboccipital triangle via condylar canal.
5. **Venous plexus of foramen ovale:** It connects cavernous sinus to pterygoid plexus of veins.
6. **Venous plexus in carotid canal:** It connects cavernous sinus to internal jugular vein.
7. **Petrosquamous sinus:** It connects transverse sinus to external jugular vein.
8. **Occipital emissary vein:** It connects confluence of sinuses with occipital vein.

Q.197. What are cells present in pituitary and their secretion.

Ans.

Anterior pituitary	*Secretion*
Gonadotropes	FSH, LH
Thyrotropes	TSH
Corticotropes	ACTH
Mammotropes	Prolactin
Somatotropes	GH
Posterior pituitary	*Secretion*
Posterior pituitary	Vasopressin (ADH) Oxytocin
Intermediate pituitary	*Secretion*
Intermediate pituitary	MSH

Q.198. What is arterial supply of pituitary gland?

Ans.

1. **Superior hypophyseal artery:** Branch of internal carotid artery.
2. **Inferior hypophyseal artery:** Branch of internal carotid artery.
3. **Portal vessels:** The anterior lobe of pituitary is supplied by long and short portal vessels. The portal vessels are continuations of the external and internal capillary plexuses formed by the two superior hypophyseal arteries at the median eminence and upper infundibulum.

Q.199. What are contents of temporal fossa?

Ans.

1. Temporalis muscle
2. Temporal fascia
3. Deep temporal vessels
4. Deep temporal nerves
5. Auriculotemporal nerve
6. Superficial temporal vessels

Q.200. What are contents of infratemporal fossa?

Ans.

1. Muscles
   a. Tendon of temporalis muscle
   b. Lateral and medial pterygoid muscles
2. Nerves
   a. Mandibular nerve and its branches
   b. Chorda tympani, branch of facial nerve
   c. Otic ganglion
3. Vessels
   a. Maxillary artery
   b. Pterygoid venous plexus

Q.201. What are contents of pterygopalatine fossa?

Ans.

1. Maxillary nerve: It reaches the fossa through the foramen rotundum over the anterior surface of root of pterygoid process.
2. Pterygopalatine ganglion and its connections.
3. Maxillary artery, 3rd part: It enters the fossa via the pterygomaxillary fissure and divides into its terminal branches.

Q.202. Name the branches of Ist part of maxillary artery?

Ans. (Fig. 1.29)

1. Deep auricular artery
2. Anterior tympanic artery
3. Middle meningeal artery
4. Accessory meningeal artery
5. Inferior alveolar artery

Q.20.3. Name the branches of 2nd part of maxillary artery?

Ans. (Fig. 1.29)

1. Deep temporal artery
2. Pterygoid branches
3. Masseteric artery
4. Buccal artery

Q. 204. Name the branches of 3rd part of maxillary artery?

Ans. (Fig. 1.29)

1. Posterior superior alveolar (dental) artery
2. Infraorbital artery
3. Greater palatine artery
4. Pharyngeal artery
5. Artery of pterygoid canal
6. Sphenopalatine artery

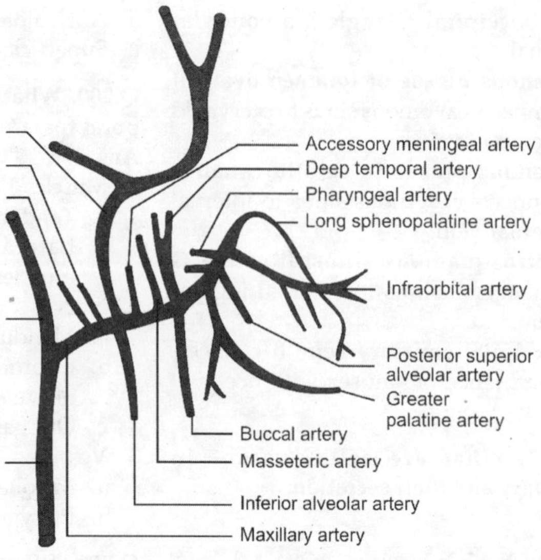

Fig. 1.29: Maxillary artery and its branches

Q.205. Name the veins forming pterygoid venous plexus?

Ans. It is the plexus of veins present over the lateral pterygoid muscle, part of plexus lies between the lateral and medial pterygoid muscles. It is formed by the following veins:

1. Sphenopalatine vein
2. Deep temporal vein
3. Pterygoid vein
4. Masseteric vein
5. Buccal vein
6. Alveolar veins
7. Greater palatine vein
8. Middle meningeal veins
9. Branches from ophthalmic vein

Q.206. Temporomandibular joint is which type of joint?

Ans. It is condylar variety of synovial joint. Anatomically there are two temporomandibular joints but physiologically they are one.

Q.207. Name the ligaments of temporomandibular joint?

Ans. They are:

1. Fibrous capsule
2. Lateral temporomandibular ligament
3. Sphenomandibular ligament
4. Stylomandibular ligament

Q.208. What is the nerve supply of temporomandibular (TM) joint?

Ans. It is supplied by branches of mandibular division of trigeminal nerve namely:

1. Auriculotemporal nerve
2. Masseteric nerve

Q.209. Why do you have articular disk in temporomandibular joint?

Ans. Articular disk is an oval fibrocartilaginous plate with a concavo-convex superior surface and a concave inferior surface, to accommodate the head of mandible. It is thickend at the periphery to form an annulus which is attached to the fibrous capsule.

Functions of articular disk of joint

1. It divides the joint cavity into two parts:
   a. Upper meniscal-temporal compartment—permits gliding movements.
   b. Lower menisco-mandibular compartment—permits rotatory as well as gliding movements.
2. It reduces the friction between the two articular surfaces. It allows free sliding movement of the condyle preventing damage due to friction. This function is at the cost of slight instability of the joint.
3. It aids in lubrication of the joint.

Q.210. What is dislocation of temporomandibular joint?

Ans. Dislocation of temporomandibular joint usually occurs when the mouth is widely open. In this position the head of mandible glides forwards and downwards and comes to lie below the articular tubercle. The joint is highly unstable and a blow on head in this position results in forward dislocation of the head of mandible. The person will not be able to close his mouth after such an injury.

Q.211. What are the boundaries of parotid bed?

Ans. Boundaries of parotid bed or retromandibular fossa are:

1. Anterior: Posterior border of ramus of mandible, laterally, masseter and medial pterygoid muscles, medially.
2. Posterior: Mastoid process, sternocleidomastoid muscle, laterally.
3. Superior: External acoustic meatus, posterior part of the temporomandibular joint.
4. Inferior: Posterior belly of digastric and stylohyoid muscles.
5. Medial: Styloid process, styloglossus, stylopharyngeus and stylohyoid muscles.

Q.212. What are structures present within parotid gland?

Ans. Structures present within the parotid gland (Fig. 1.30)

1. Facial nerve and its branches:
2. Retromandibular vein
3. External carotid artery
4. Deep parotid lymph nodes

Q.213. What is parasympathetic nerve supply of parotid gland?

Ans. The preganglionic fibers arise from inferior salivatory nucleus and pass successively through the glossopharyngeal nerve, tympanic branch of glossopharyngeal nerve, tympanic plexus and lesser petrosal nerve to relay in the otic ganglion. Postganglionic fibers arise from the cells of the ganglion and pass through auriculotemporoal nerve to supply the parotid gland. It is secretomotor and results in secretion of watery fluid (Fig. 1.31).

Q.214. What is sympathetic nerve supply of parotid glands?

Ans. It is derived from the sympathetic plexus around the external carotid artery which is formed by the postganglionic fibers from superior cervical sympathetic ganglion. It is secretomotor and results in production of mucus rich sticky secretion. It is also vasomotor to the gland (Fig. 1.31).

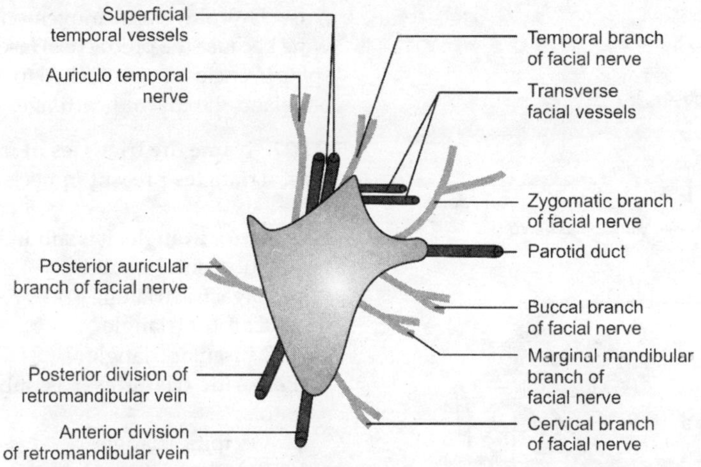

Fig. 1.30: Parotid gland and structures present in it

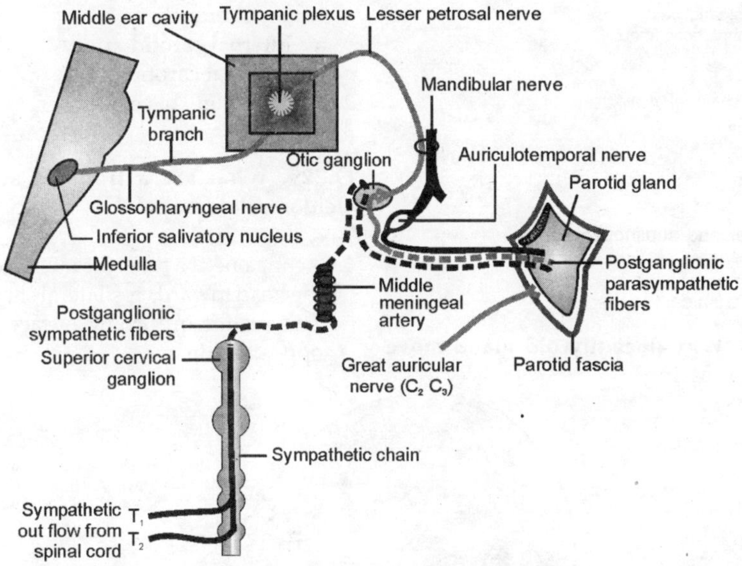

Fig. 1.31: Nerve supply of parotid gland

Q.215. What is sensory nerve supply of parotid gland?

Ans. It is through following nerves:

1. From auriculotemporal nerve
2. From great auricular nerve
3. C_2 is sensory to parotid fascia

Q.216. What is mumps?

Ans. Mumps is a viral infection which has special affinity for the parotid glands and results in swollen and painful glands. Pain is severe as the gland is surrounded by a tough capsule. Mastication is also painful due to inflammation of the glenoid process of gland which is closely related to the tempromandibular joint. Mumps is self-limiting and requires only supportive care. Rarely it can lead to complications like bronchitis, orchitis and pancreatitis.

Q.217. Describe the treatment of a parotid abscess?

Ans. Infection of parotid gland generally is a consequence of retrograde bacterial infection from mouth through the parotid duct. Severe infection leading to an abscess is drained by giving a horizontal incision over it. A vertical incision is avoided as it can lead to injury to branches of the facial nerve.

Q.218. What is nerve supply of submandibular gland?

Ans. Nerve supply of submandibular gland (Fig. 1.32):

1. **Parasympathetic:** Preganglionic fibers arise from superior salivatory nucleus. They pass successively through the facial nerve, chorda tympani nerve, lingual nerve and relay into the submandibular ganglion. Postganglionic fibers arise from cells of the ganglion and directly supply the gland. It is secretomotor and causes secretion of watery fluid.
2. **Sympathetic:** Is derived from the sympathetic plexus around facial artery formed by postganglionic fibers from superior cervical sympathetic ganglion. It is secretomotor and results in secretion of mucus rich fluid. It is also vasomotor.
3. **Sensory:** Lingual nerve.

Q.219. What is nerve supply of sublingual gland?

Ans. It is same as submandibular gland except postganglionic parasympathetic secretomotor fibers are carried by lingual nerve.

Q.220. Name the tributaries of external jugular vein?

Ans. The tributories of external jugular vein are:

1. Posterior division of retromandibular vein
2. Posterior auricular vein
3. Anterior jugular vein
4. Posterior external jugular vein
5. Transverse cervical vein
6. Suprascapular vein
7. It communicates with internal jugular vein by and oblique jugular vein

Q.221. What is cutaneous nerve supply of neck?

Ans. Cutaneous nerver supply of neck is derived from the following branches of cervical plexus:

1. Lesser occipital nerve (C_2)
2. Great auricular nerve ($C_{2,3}$)
3. Transverse cutaneous nerve of neck ($C_{2,3}$)

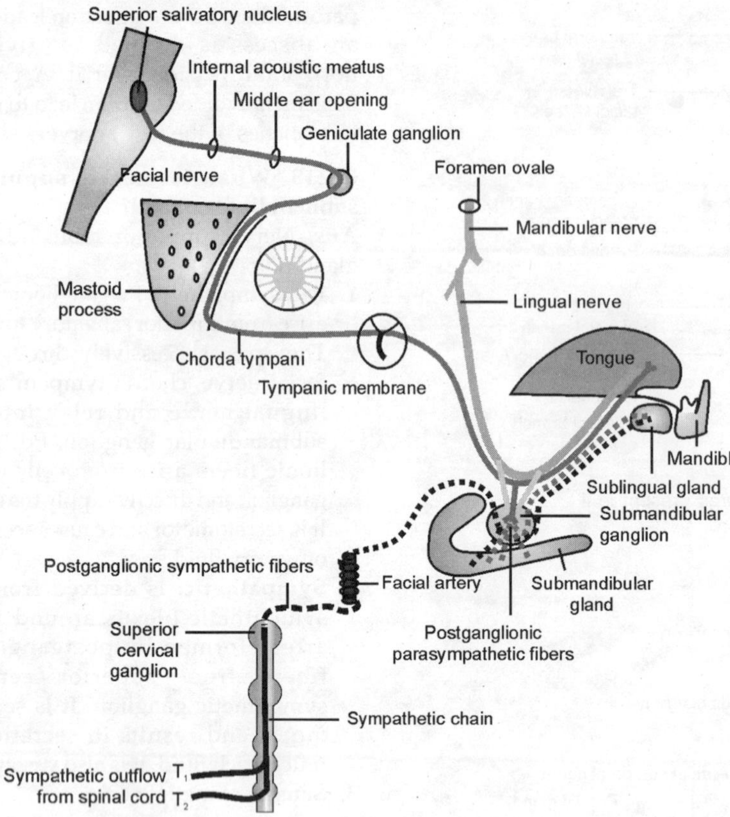

Fig. 1.32: Nerve supply of submandibular and sublingual glands

4. Supraclavicular nerve ($C_{3,4}$)
5. Medial branches of dorsal rami of $C_{3,4,5}$ spinal nerves

Q.222. What are layers of deep fascia of neck?

Ans. It consists of three layers, from exterior to interior
1. Investing layer
2. Pretracheal layer
3. Prevertebral layer

Q.223. What is the extent of carotid sheath?

Ans. It extends from the base of skull above to the arch of aorta below.

Q. 224. What are contents of carotid sheath?

Ans.
1. Common carotid artery in lower part and internal carotid artery in upper part
2. Internal jugular vein
3. Vagus nerve

Q.225. Which nerve is embedded in anterior wall of carotid sheath?

Ans. Ansa cervicalis.

Q.226. Why does thyroid gland move on swallowing?

Ans. Thyroid gland moves on swallowing because the pretracheal fascia which splits to enclose it, is attached to the hyoid bone and the thyroid cartilage.

Q.227. Name the triangles of neck?

Ans. Triangles present in neck are (Fig. 1.33):
1. **Anterior triangle:** It is subdivided into
   a. Submental triangle
   b. Digastric triangle
   c. Carotid triangle
   d. Muscular triangle
2. **Posterior triangle:** It is subdivided into
   a. Occipital triangle
   b. Subclavian triangle

Q.228. What are the contents of carotid triangle?

Ans. The contents of carotid triangle are:
1. Common carotid artery with its terminal branches
   a. Internal carotid artery
   b. External carotid artery
2. Internal jugular vein
3. Occipital vessels

Q.229. What are actions of sternocleidomastoid muscle?

Ans.
1. Acting one at a time, the muscle draws the head towards ipsilateral shoulder. This results in turning of face to the opposite side.

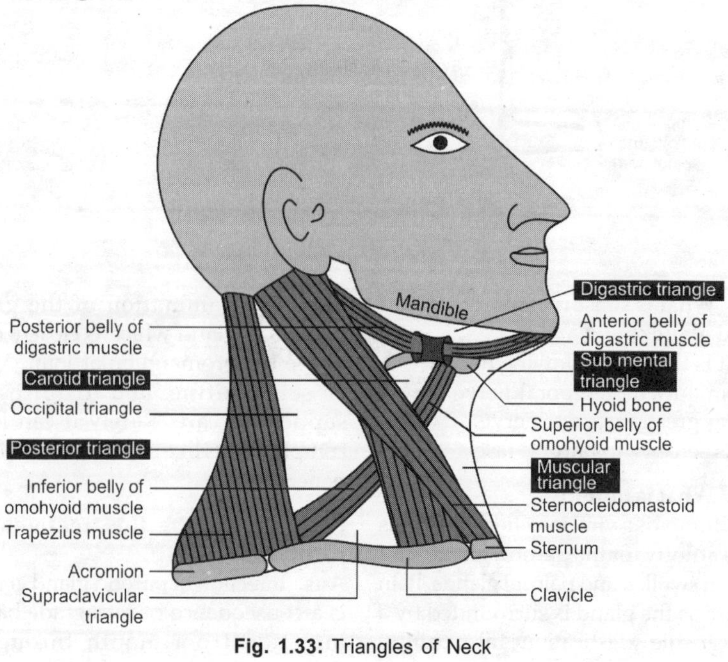

Fig. 1.33: Triangles of Neck

2. Flexion of neck is brought about when muscles of both sides act together. Along with action of longus colli, they bring about flexion of cervical part of vertebral column.
3. They aid in elevation of thorax during inspiration, when the head is fixed.
4. Posterior most fibers of both muscles causes extension of neck to peeping over the crowd.

Q.230. Name the branches of external carotid artery?

Ans. The external carotid artery gives 8 branches, (Fig. 1.34):

1. Ascending pharyngeal artery
2. Superior thyroid artery
3. Lingual artery
4. Facial artery
5. Occipital artery
6. Posterior auricular artery
7. Maxillary artery
8. Superficial temporal artery

Q.231. Name the branches of lingual artery?

Ans. Branches of lingual artery are:

1. **Suprahyoid branch:** It arises from the first part and anastomoses with its fellow of opposite side.
2. **Dorsal lingual branches:** These are usually two in number and arise from the 2nd part. They supply the dorsum of tongue and the tonsil.
3. **Sublingual artery:** It is given off from the 3rd part and supplies the sublingual gland.

Q.232. Name the branches of facial artery?

Ans.

1. Branches from cervical part (in the neck)
   a. Ascending palatine artery
   b. Tonsillar artery (main artery of tonsil)
   c. Glandular branches to supply the submandibular gland
   d. Submental artery
2. Branches from the facial part (in the face)
   a. Inferior labial artery
   b. Superior labial artery
   c. Lateral nasal artery
   d. Angular artery
   e. Small unnamed branches: These are small and arise from the posterior aspect of the artery.

Q.233. Name the branches of occipital artery?

Ans.

1. Sternomastoid branches
2. Mastoid branches
3. Meningeal branches
4. Muscular branches
5. Auricular branch
6. Descending branches
7. Occipital branches

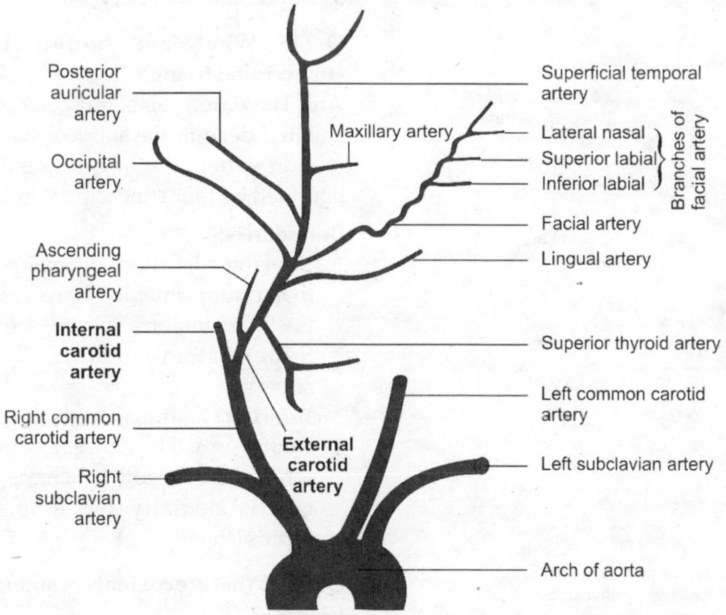

Fig. 1.34: Branches of external carotid artery

Q.234. Enumerate the parts of internal carotid artery?

Ans. It is divided into four parts:

1. Cervical part
2. Petrous part
3. Cavernous part
4. Cerebral part

Q235. Name the branches of cerebral part of internal carotid artery?

Ans.

1. Ophthalmic artery
2. Anterior choroidal artery
3. Posterior communicating artery
4. Anterior cerebral artery
5. Middle cerebral artery

Q.236. Name the tributaries of internal jugular vein?

Ans.

1. Inferior petrosal sinus
2. Pharyngeal veins
3. Common facial vein
4. Lingual vein
5. Superior thyroid vein
6. Middle thyroid vein
7. Occipital vein

Q.237. What are the contents of occipital triangle (part of posterior triangle)?

Ans. Contents (from above downwards):

1. Occipital artery at apex
2. Spinal part of accessory nerve
3. Four cutaneous branches of cervical plexus of nerves
   a. Lesser occipital
   b. Great auricular
   c. Transverse cutaneous nerve of neck
   d. Supraclavicular
4. Muscular branches of C_3 and C_4 nerves
5. Upper part of brachial plexus
6. Dorsal scapular nerve
7. Superficial cervical vessels, branches of vertebral vessels
8. Lymph nodes

Q.238. What are the contents of subclavian or supraclavicular triangle?

Ans. Contents of supraclavicular triangle are:

1. Supraclavicular nerves
2. Trunks of brachial plexus of nerves with their branches:
   a. Dorsal scapular nerve
   b. Long thoracic nerve
   c. Nerve to subclavius

3. 3rd part of subclavian artery
4. Subclavian vein, lies behind the clavicle
5. Suprascapular vessels
6. External jugular vein
7. Supraclavicular lymph nodes

Q.239. Name the structures that pierce the fascial roof of posterior triangle?

Ans. Structures that pierces the fascial roof of posterior triangle are:

1. The cutaneous branches of cervical plexus. These are:
   a. Lesser occipital nerve (C_2)
   b. Great auricular nerve (C_2, C_3)
   c. Transverse cervical cutaneous nerve (C_2, C_3)
   d. Supraclavicular nerve (C_3, C_4)
2. External jugular vein: It pierces the deep fascia from without to drain into the subclavian vein.

Q.240. What is the root value of cervical plexus?

Ans. The plexus is formed by the interconnection of ventral rami of upper four cervical nerves, C_1, C_2, C_3 and C_4.

Q.241. Name the branches of cervical plexus?

Ans. Branches of cervical plexus are (Fig. 1.35):

Superficial cutaneous branches

1. Lesser occipital nerve, (C_2)
2. Great auricular nerve, ($C_{2, 3}$)
3. Transverse cervical nerve, ($C_{2, 3}$)
4. Supraclavicular nerve, ($C_{3, 4}$)

Deep muscular branches: They supply the muscles directly or indirectly via communicating branches:

1. Phrenic nerve, ($C_{3, 4, 5}$): This supplies the diaphragm.
2. Descendens cervicalis nerve, ($C_{2, 3}$): This joins with descendans hypoglossi to form ansa cervicalis in front of the carotid sheath. It supplies sternohyoid, sternothyroid and inferior belly of omohyoid.
3. Branches from C_1 communicates with hypoglossal nerve to supply thyrohyoid, geniohyoid and superior belly of omohyoid muscles.
4. $C_{2,3,4}$ communicate with the spinal root of accessory nerve to supply sternocleidomastoid (C_2).

Q.242. Name the branches of subclavian artery?

Ans. The subclavian artery gives 5 branches (Fig. 1.36):

1. **From first part**
   a. Vertebral artery
   b. Internal thoracic artery
   c. Thyrocervical trunk
   d. Costocervical trunk (on left side only)
2. **From second part**
   a. Costocervical trunk (on right side only)
3. **From third part**
   a. Dorsal scapular artery

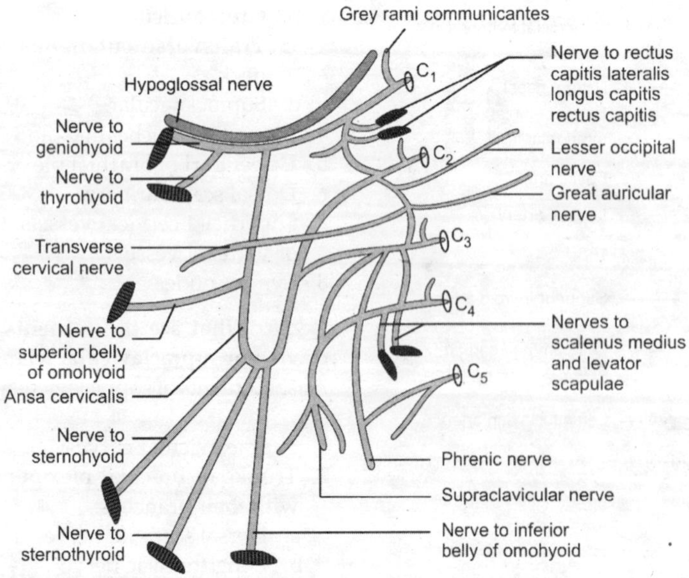

Fig. 1.35: Cervical plexus and its branches

Q.243. Name the branches of vertebral artery?

Ans. Branches of vertebral artery are:

1. **In the neck**
   a. Spinal branches, which enter the vertebral canal through intervertebral foramen to supply the upper 5 or 6 cervical segments of the spinal cord.
   b. Muscular branches, they arise from the 3rd part of vertebral artery and supply muscles of suboccipital triangle.
2. **In the cranial cavity**
   a. Meningeal branches, they supply meninges of posterior cranial fossa.
   b. Posterior spinal artery (sometimes it may arise from posterior inferior cerebellar artery).
   c. Posterior inferior cerebellar artery (largest branch of the vertebral artery).
   d. Anterior spinal artery
   e. Medullar branches supply the medulla.

Q.244. Name the branches of thyrocervical trunk?

Ans. The thyrocervical trunk is very small and divides almost at once into three branches:

1. Inferior thyroid artery: Branches:
2. Superficial cervical artery
3. Suprascapular artery

Q.245. What are boundaries of suboccipital triangle?

Ans. These are a pair of muscular triangles situated deep in the suboccipital region one on either side of midline and are bounded by four suboccipital muscles.

Boundaries:

1. **Superomedial:** Rectus capitis posterior major, supplemented by rectus capitis posterior minor.
2. **Superolateral:** Obliquus capitis superior
3. **Inferior:** Obliquus capitis inferior
4. **Roof:** Formed by dense fibrous tissue which is covered by semispinalis capitis medially and longissimus capitis laterally.

Q.246. What are contents of suboccipital triangle?

Ans.

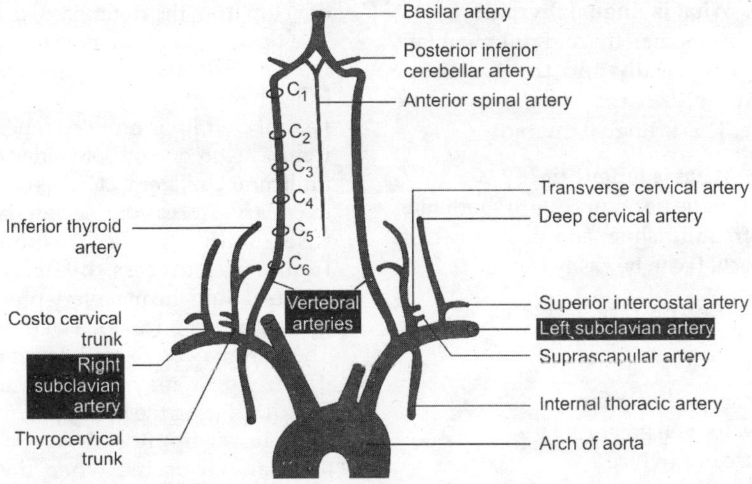

Fig. 1.36: Subclavian arteries and their branches

1. 3rd part of vertebral artery.
2. Dorsal ramus of C_1 (suboccipital nerve)
3. Suboccipital plexus of veins

Q.247. What is vestibule of mouth?

Ans. The vestibule of mouth is a narrow space that lies outside the teeth and gums and inside the lips and cheeks.

Q.248. What opens in vestibule of mouth?

Ans. The parotid duct opens into the lateral wall of vestibule opposite the crown of upper second molar tooth.

Q.249. What are the types of mucosa present in oral cavity?

Ans. Mucosal lining of oral cavity is of three types:

1. **Lining mucosa:** It lines most of oral cavity and is made up of non-keratinized stratified squamous epithelium
2. **Masticatory mucosa:** It is present over alveolar processes and is made up of keratinized stratified squamous epithelium
3. **Specialized mucosa:** It is present over dorsum of tongue and forms lingual papillae

Q.250. What are the parts of tooth?

Ans. Parts of tooth are (Fig. 1.37):

1. Pulp cavity
2. Dentine
3. Enamel
4. Cementum
5. Periodontal ligament or membrane

Q.251. What are timings of eruption of deciduous teeth?

Ans. The age of eruption is as follows:

Teeth	*Time of eruption*
Lower central incisors	6 months
Upper central incisors	7 months
Lateral incisors	8–9 months
First molar	12 months (1 year)
Canines	18 months (1 ½ year)

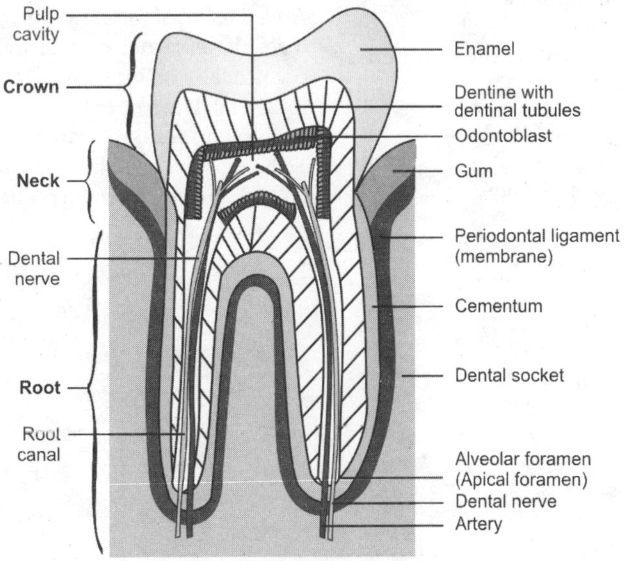

Fig. 1.37: Structure of tooth

Q.252. Why is osteomyelitis, i.e. inflammation of bone more common after extraction of lower teeth?

Ans. Sometimes extraction of a tooth leads to osteomyelitis of the jaw. It usually occurs in the lower jaw and not in the upper jaw. This is because, the lower jaw is supplied by a single inferior alveolar artery. Therefore, damage to this artery during extraction produces bone necrosis. The upper jaw on the other hand receives segmental supply by 3 arteries namely, posterior superior, middle superior and anterior superior alveolar arteries. Therefore ischemia does not occur following injury to an individual artery.

Q.253. What is dental caries?

Ans. It is the disintegration of one of the calcified structures covering the pulp cavity. The most important cause is inadequate oral hygeine. It leads to inflammation and pain in the involved tooth due to exposure of the pulp cavity.

Q.254. What are functions of tongue?
Ans.
1. Receives bolus of food
2. Mastication (chewing of food)
3. Deglutition (swallowing of food)
4. Peripheral apparatus of taste
5. Speech
6. Facial expression
7. Paste postage stamp
8. Pattern of papillae has medicolegal importance

Q.255. What is the sensory supply of tongue?
Ans. Sensory supply of tongue is obtained from (Fig. 1.38):
1. **Lingual nerve:** Receives general sensation from anterior 2/3rd of the tongue.
2. **Chorda tympani:** Receives taste sensations from anterior 2/3rd except from vallate papillae.
3. **Glossopharyngeal nerve**
   - Conveys all general sensations from posterior 1/3rd of the tongue.
   - Carries taste sensation from vallate papillae.
4. **Internal laryngeal branch of superior laryngeal nerve** conveys taste sensation from posterior most part of tongue and vallecula.

Q.256. What is aglossia?
Ans. Aglossia is complete absence of the tongue, due to total developmental failure.

Q.257. What is bifid tongue?
Ans. Bifid tongue occurs due to non fusion of lingual swellings.

Q.258. What is lingual thyroid?
Ans. The median thyroid rudiment fails to grow caudally and thyroid tissue persists within the substance of the tongue. This is lingual thyroid.

Q.259. What is tongue tie?
Ans. Tongue tie occurs due to shortening of the frenulum linguae and can interfere in speech. It can be easily excised.

Q.260. Enumerate muscles of soft palate?
Ans.
1. Tensor veli palatini
2. Levator veli palatini
3. Musculus uvulae
4. Palatoglossus
5. Palatopharyngeus

Q.261. Which muscle of palate help in opening the auditory tube?
Ans. Tensor veli palatini.

Q.262. What is the result of paralysis of muscles of soft palate?
Ans. Paralysis of muscles of soft palate due to lesion of vagus nerve produces
1. Nasal regurgitation of liquids
2. Nasal twang in voice
3. Flattening of the palatal arch on the side of lesion
4. Deviation of uvula, opposite to the side of lesion

Q.263. What is cleft lip?
Ans. Fusion of the various processes that form the external part of the face may occasionally be incomplete and give rise to cleft lip. It can be of the following types:
1. **Cleft upper lip:** It can be median cleft lip or lateral cleft lip. Median cleft lip is rare and occurs if the philtrum fails to develop from the frontonasal process. The upper lip of hare normally has a median cleft, therefore this defect is called hare-lip.
   Lateral cleft lip is more common and it may be on one or both sides of the philtrum. Unilateral cleft lip occurs if maxillary process of one side fails to fuse with the corresponding frontonasal process. Bilateral cleft occurs if both the maxillary processes fail to fuse with frontonasal process.
   The cleft may be a small defect in the upper lip or may extend into the nostril splitting the upper jaw.
2. **Cleft lower lip:** It is always median and rare. It occurs when the two mandibular processes do not fuse with each other. The defect usually extends into the lower jaw.

Q.264. What is macrostomia?
Ans. Macrostomia or big mouth occurs due to inadequate fusion of the mandibular and maxillary processes with each other. The lack of fusion may be unilateral. This leads to the formation of lateral facial cleft.

Q.265. What is microstomia?
Ans. Too much fusion of mandibular and maxillary processes may result in the small mouth or microstomia.

Q.266. What is the cleft palate?
Ans. The defective fusion of various segments of the palate gives rise to clefts in the palate. These vary considerably in degree, leading to varieties of cleft palate.

Q.267. Enumerate the openings present in lateral wall of nose?
Ans. Openings in the lateral wall of the nose (Fig. 1.39):

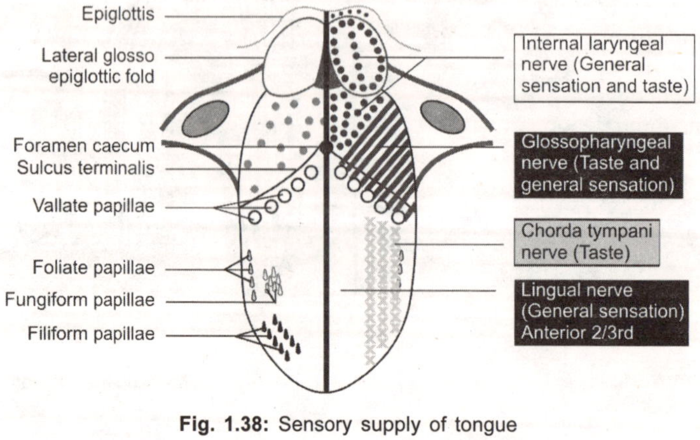

Fig. 1.38: Sensory supply of tongue

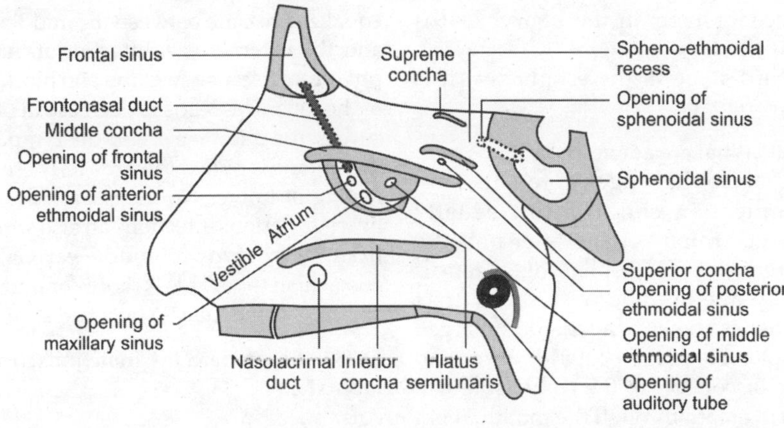

Fig. 1.39: Openings in lateral wall of nose

Site	*Opening/Openings*
Sphenoethmoidal recess	Opening of sphenoidal air sinus
Superior meatus	Openings of posterior ethmoidal air sinuses
Middle meatus	
a. On bulla ethmoidalis	Openings of middle ethmoidal air sinus
b. In hiatus semilunaris	
– Anterior part	Opening of frontal air sinus
– Middle part	Opening of anterior ethmoidal air sinus
– Posterior part	Opening of maxillary air sinus
Inferior meatus	Opening of nasolacrimal duct (at the junction of anterior 1/3rd and posterior 2/3rd)

Q.268. What is Little's area and what is its clinical importance?

Ans. The area on the antero-inferior part of the nasal septum is highly vascular. In this area the septal branches of anterior ethmoidal, sphenopalatine, greater palatine and superior labial arteries anastomose to form a plexus known as Kesselbach's plexus. This area is named as the Little's area and is the most common site of epistaxis or bleeding from nose in children.

Q.269. What is deviated nasal septum?

Ans. The central septum of the nose may be deviated in some to the right or to the left side leading to varying degrees of obstruction of the respective nasal cavity. The deviation commonly involves the cartilaginous part and occasionally the bony part of septum. It can lead to recurrent attacks of nasal blockage and sinusitis. This condition is treated surgically by submucous resection of the deviated part of the septum.

Q.270. Where do you find olfactory epithelium?

Ans. Olfactory epithelium is present in relation to the roof of nasal cavity over the nasal bones and superior conchae. It is present over an area of 2.5 cm^2 and is supplied by olfactory nerves.

Q.271. Maxillary hiatus is reduced in size by 4 bones, what are these bones?

Ans.

1. Unicate process of ethmoid, from above.
2. Descending process of lacrimal bone, from above.
3. Ethmoidal process of inferior nasal concha, from below.
4. Perpendicular plate of palatine bone from behind.

Q.272. What is the clinical importance of maxillary sinus?

Ans. Maxillary sinus is the commonest site of infection amongst all sinuses. The infection is called maxillary sinusitis. This infection can occur from the following sources

1. Infection in the nose
2. Caries of upper molar teeth
3. Being the most dependant part it acts as a secondary reservoir of pus from frontal air sinuses through fronto-nasal duct and hiatus semilunaris.

The opening of the sinus is unfortunately present in the upper part of its medial wall. This results in inefficient drainage and persistence of infection.

Q.273. What are methods of surgical drainage of maxillary air sinus?

Ans. Surgical drainage of maxillary sinus may be performed by following ways:

1. **Endoscopic sinus surgery**
2. **Antral puncture** by passing a trocar and cannula in the inferior meatus in an outward and backward direction to create a separate opening in the medial wall of the sinus at a lower level.
3. **Caldwell Luc operation:** In this surgery a fenestra is created in the anterior wall of sinus above the canine fossa through the gingivo-labial fold.

Q.274. What is Waldeyer's lymphatic ring?

Ans. It consists of collections of lymphoid tissue in the submucosal layer of the wall of air and food passages around their commencement. The lymph nodules are arranged in a ring like pattern, from posterior to anterior forming the Walderyer's lymphatic ring. It is made up of the following (Fig. 1.40):

1. Pharyngeal (nasopharyngeal) tonsils
2. Tubal tonsils
3. Palatine tonsils
4. Lingual tonsil

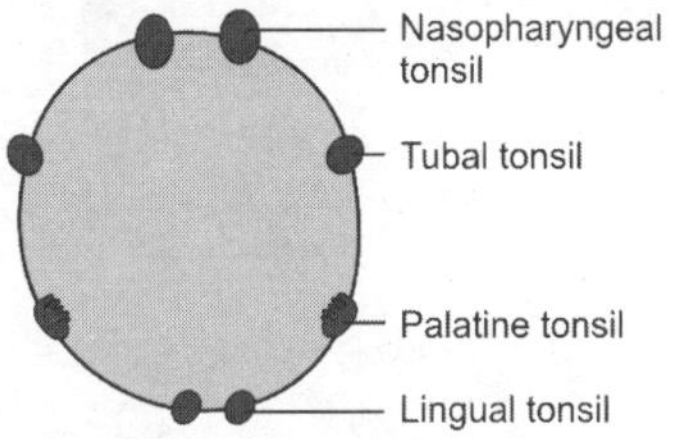

Fig. 1.40: Waldeyer's ring

Q.275. Enumerate the structures passing above superior constrictor of pharynx?

Ans. Between the base of skull and upper concave border of superior constrictor muscle of pharynx lies the sinus of Morgagni. It gives passage to (Fig. 1.41)

1. Auditory tube
2. Levator palati muscle

3. Ascending palatine artery
4. Palatine branch of ascending pharyngeal artery

Q.276. Name the structures passing between superior and middle constrictors of pharynx?

Ans. (Fig. 1.41)
1. Stylopharyngeus muscle
2. Glossopharyngeal nerve

Q.277. Name the structures passing between middle and inferior constrictors of pharynx?

Ans. (Fig. 1.41)
1. Internal laryngeal nerve
2. Superior laryngeal vessels

Q.278. Name the structures passing below inferior constrictor muscle of pharynx, in the tracheoesophageal groove?

Ans. (Fig. 1.41)
1. Recurrent laryngeal nerve
2. Inferior laryngeal vessels

Q.279. What are stages of deglutition?

Ans. Deglutition is a process by which the food is transferred from the mouth to the stomach. It consists of three successive stages:
1. First stage, in the mouth. It is voluntary
2. Second stage, in the pharynx. It is involuntary
3. Third stage in the esophagus, it is involuntary

Q.280. What are adenoids?

Ans. Nasopharyngeal tonsils are prominent in children but usually undergo atrophy at and after puberty. Enlargement of nasopharyngeal tonsils usually due to upper respiratory tract infection is known as adenoids. Enlarged adenoids block the posterior nares and cause discomfort to the child as he will have to breath through the mouth. It is a common cause of snoring in children.

Q.281. What is the clinical importance of piriform fossa?

Ans. Piriform fossa is a depressed area where occasionally the ingested food particles can get stuck. If adequate care is not taken during the removal of a foreign body especially any hard structure like fish bones, it may damage the internal laryngeal nerve leading to anesthesia in the supraglottic part of the larynx.

Q.282. What is the clinical significance of the eustachian tube?

Ans. The eustachian tube extends from middle ear to nasopharynx and helps to equalize pressure between the middle ear and the external ear. Infection in nasopharynx can cause swelling and blockage of the tube. This leads to decrease in pressure in the middle ear and the tympanic membrane is pulled towards it. There is a feeling of fullness in the ear and loss of hearing. Serious infection can also spread from the pharynx to middle ear via the eustachian tube. This is more common in children as the tube is short and straight.

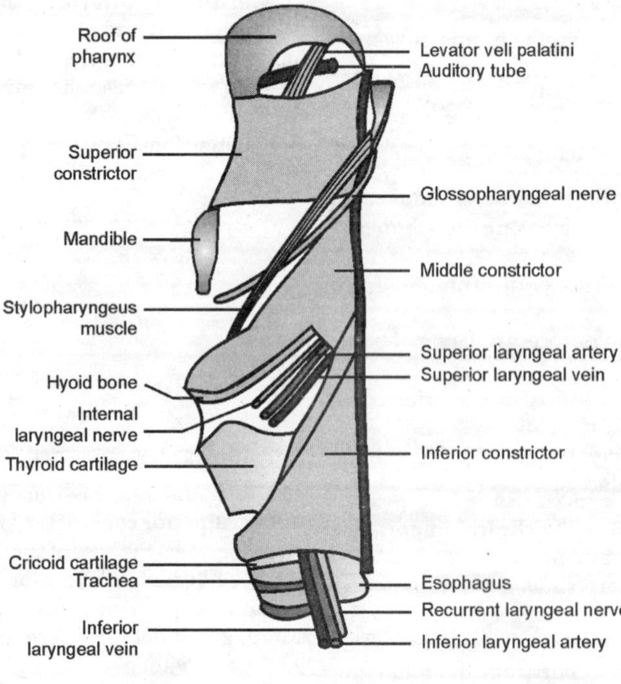

Fig. 1.41: Strctures passing between constrictors of pharynx

Q.283. Enumerate intrinsic muscles of larynx?

Ans.
1. Oblique arytenoid
2. Aryepiglotticus
3. Posterior cricoarytenoid
4. Lateral cricoarytenoid
5. Transverse arytenoid
6. Cricothyroid
7. Thyroarytenoid
8. Vocalis
9. Thyroepiglotticus

Q.284. Name the adductors of vocal cords?

Ans.
1. Lateral cricoarytenoids
2. Transverse arytenoids

Q.285. Name the abductor of vocal cords?

Ans. Posterior cricoarytenoids.

Q.286. Name the tensors of vocal cords?

Ans.
1. Cricothyroids
2. Vocalis

Q.287. What is sensory supply of larynx above glottis?

Ans. Internal laryngeal nerve.

Q.288. Enumerate cartilages present in larynx?

Ans. Larynx is made up of three paired and three unpaired cartilages.

Paired cartilages	*Unpaired cartilages*
They are small and comprise of	*They are large and comprise of (from above downwards)*
1. Arytenoid	1. Epiglottis
2. Corniculate	2. Thyroid
3. Cuneiform	3. Cricoid

Q.289. Enumerate the nerves supplying external ear or pinna?